AF760276

Radio-Frequency Human Exposure Assessment

To Corinne, Romain and Thibaut

FOCUS SERIES

Series Editor Pierre-Noël Favennec

Radio-Frequency Human Exposure Assessment

From Deterministic to Stochastic Methods

Joe Wiart

iSTE

WILEY

First published 2016 in Great Britain and the United States by ISTE Ltd and John Wiley & Sons, Inc.

Apart from any fair dealing for the purposes of research or private study, or criticism or review, as permitted under the Copyright, Designs and Patents Act 1988, this publication may only be reproduced, stored or transmitted, in any form or by any means, with the prior permission in writing of the publishers, or in the case of reprographic reproduction in accordance with the terms and licenses issued by the CLA. Enquiries concerning reproduction outside these terms should be sent to the publishers at the undermentioned address:

ISTE Ltd
27-37 St George's Road
London SW19 4EU
UK

www.iste.co.uk

John Wiley & Sons, Inc.
111 River Street
Hoboken, NJ 07030
USA

www.wiley.com

© ISTE Ltd 2016
The rights of Joe Wiart to be identified as the author of this work have been asserted by him in accordance with the Copyright, Designs and Patents Act 1988.

Library of Congress Control Number: 2016930390

British Library Cataloguing-in-Publication Data
A CIP record for this book is available from the British Library
ISBN 978-1-84821-856-7

Contents

Preface

"Out of clutter, find simplicity. From discord, find harmony. In the middle of difficulty lies opportunity".

Albert EINSTEIN

Approximately 6 billion humans are nowadays using a mobile phone. Depending on the country, these wireless phones are known as "handy", "cellular", "mobile", "smartphone", etc. Like electricity, the car and television, they have changed our way of life. Nowadays, they play an important role in our daily life.

Before the 1990s, mobiles phones were, for the most part, bulky and only used by a small number of people. The 1990s saw an increasing and tremendous use of wireless systems and the democratization of this means of communication.

The use of electromagnetic waves for wireless communication is not new: Marconi patented the first wireless communication system in 1897. For a long time, firefighters, hospitals and police used radio waves to communicate but it took until the 1980s to lay down the foundations of the current wireless telephone networks that today allow hundreds of millions of people to make calls, download information, surf the Internet, etc.

To enable communication between millions of phones, computers and, more recently, tablets, millions of access points, i.e. base station antennas, have been deployed globally (tens of thousand in France). Small cell technology and the Internet of Things, with billions of connected objects, will reinforce this trend.

Despite (or because) of this proximity, electromagnetic radiation emitted by the antennas raises many questions and concerns about the possible health effects of these devices. These radiofrequency waves emit non-ionizing radiation. These waves are not mutagenic, but if the energy carried is too high, they are capable of inducing adverse health effects. To protect people from these possible effects, standards have been established. The World Health Organization (WHO) recommended that biological, biomedical and epidemiological studies be conducted to verify that no health effects are caused below the exposure levels inducing thermal effects. These compliance checks and biomedical research require a quantification of human exposure. This is the purpose of dosimetry.

Dosimetry is a relatively new domain in electromagnetism. It is fundamental for assessing the specific absorption rate (SAR) and the strength of electric and magnetic fields in view of exposure quantification and compliance tests. This book introduces the experimental, numerical and statistical methods and models that have been developed between 1995 and 2015 to improve the assessment of human radiofrequency exposure.

In 2009, I cofounded with Isabelle Bloch, from Telecom ParisTech, and Christian Person, from Telecom Bretagne, the WHIST Lab that is the common lab of Orange and the Institut Mines Telecom. Since 2015, I am in charge of the Chair "Caractérisation, Modélisation et Maîtrise of the RF exposure" at Telecom ParisTech.

This book is based not only on the works performed in these structures but also on my lectures at UPMC (University Pierre & Marie Curie), UPEM (University Paris EST Marne la vallée), Telecom Bretagne and Telecom ParisTech. It takes into account the research carried out with colleagues (Christian, Man Fai, Azedine, Hamid, Emmanuelle, Nadege, Isabelle, Christian, Zwi) and students (Stephane, David, Stephanie, Naila, Jessica, Zaher, Tongning, Aimad, Amal, Majorie, Anis, Yuanyuan, Pierric, etc.). It also takes advantage of works carried out in various international collaborative research projects funded by RNRT, ANR, ANSES and FP7 between 1995 and 2015. This book consists of three chapters. The first deals with human RF exposure and wireless communication system; the second discusses computational electromagnetic applied to human exposure assessment. The third introduces a very new domain – stochastic dosimetry. This conclusion describes the recent works performed to develop and adapt statistical methods to numerical exposure assessment.

Joe WIART
January 2016

1

Human RF Exposure and Communication Systems

"Something is not just because it is law. But it must be law because it is just".

MONTESQUIEU

1.1. Introduction

Over the past 30 years, wireless communication systems have been increasingly used in our daily lives (see Figure 1.1). Worldwide, cellular phone users are more than 6 billion and mobile subscriptions will reach 9.3 billion in 2019, with more than 5.6 billion using smartphones (Figure 1.1). The versatile use of new smart mobile phones and tablets, the development of home wireless LANs as well as the emergence of pervasive wireless communication systems, such as machine-to-machine, are strengthening this tendency. At the end of 2013, the mobile broadband subscription was 2 billion, which is expected to reach 8 billion by 2019 (3G technology at 4.8 billion and 4G at 2.6 billion). By 2018, the global mobile data traffic will increase nearly 11-fold. Twenty-six billion communication devices will be on the Internet of Things by 2020, with a large proportion of these being wireless.

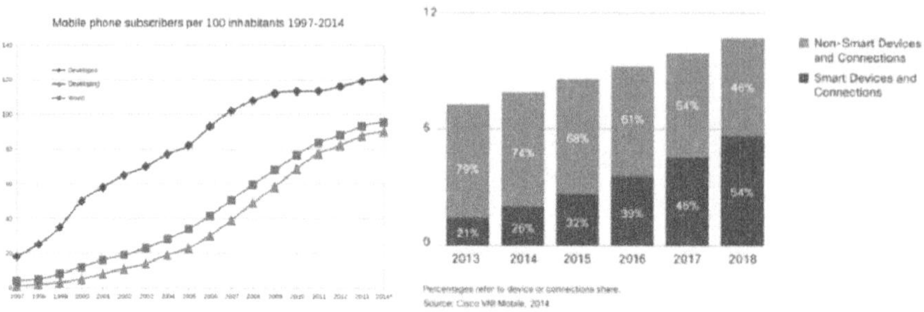

Figure 1.1. *Mobile phone subscriber's progression (left) [ICT 14]; number of devices versus years (right) [CIS 15]. For a color version of the figure, see www.iste.co.uk/wiart/radiofrequency.zip*

Despite the increasing use of wireless communications, public concerns about the possible health impacts of exposure to the *radiofrequency* (RF) *electromagnetic field* (EMF) have appeared, even if no risk has been proven to date.

In this context, the monitoring and management of EMF exposure has become a key question. Based on scientific knowledge, international organizations, such as the International Commission on Non-Ionizing Radio Protection (ICNIRP) and the Institute of Electrical and Electronics Engineers (IEEE), have established limits to protect the public against known health effects associated with EMF exposure [ICN 98, IEE 05].

In Europe, a council recommendation, based on ICNIRP guidelines and adopted in 1999, provides legal framework for the limitation of the exposure of the general public to EMFs. Equipment that intentionally emits or receives radiowaves for the purpose of radio communication has to comply with the Radio and Telecommunications Terminal Equipment (R&TTE) European Directive [DIR 14]. This directive will be replaced in 2016 by a new directive, 2014/53/EU [EU 99] (known as the Radio Equipment Directive), but the main objectives are similar. They aim to put equipment and devices onto the market and into service that satisfy the essential requirements imposed by the European Council [ECR 99].

1.2. Metric and limits relative to human exposure

1.2.1. *Human RF exposure and specific absorption rate*

The EMF induced by an RF source S is composed of an electric $\{E\}$ and a magnetic field $\{H\}$ that are governed by the Maxwell equations. In the RF domain, E and H are highly correlated. Close to the source, in the "near field", the relationship between E and H can be complex since the phase and polarization of the electric and the magnetic fields can vary with location. Far from the source, in the "far field", the EMF has, locally, a structure of a plane wave. In this case, E and H are orthogonal and the relationship between them is given by equation [1.1], where η is the free space impedance equal to 377 Ω.

$$\text{test}\frac{|\boldsymbol{E}|}{|\boldsymbol{H}|} = \boldsymbol{\eta} \qquad [1.1]$$

In the "far field", the incident power density, linked to the Poynting vector, is given by [1.2]:

$$\mathcal{P} = \frac{|\boldsymbol{E}|^2}{\eta} \qquad [1.2]$$

The human exposure to an RF-EMF is quantified through the specific absorption rate (SAR) that is the ratio of the electromagnetic power absorbed (watts) by tissues to the mass (kg) of these tissues [1.3]:

$$\text{SAR}=\frac{\text{absorbed power in volume V}}{\text{mass of the volume V}} \qquad [1.3]$$

The SAR is often averaged over the whole body or over a specific organ. The IEEE and ICNIRP standards, which have been established to limit human exposure to EMFs, use the whole body SAR (i.e. SAR averaged over the whole body). They also use the maximum SAR averaged over a mass of 10 or 1 g. In this case, the objective is to estimate the maximum SAR over a continuous volume of tissue having a mass of 1 or 10 g. The shape of the volume depends on the standard: IEEE recommends a cube shape, while ICNIRP prefers continuous tissues.

The electromagnetic energy deposited in tissues included in a volume V can be estimated through the electric field or the measurement of the rise in temperature. The first approach explains the conductivity, whereas the second approach needs information on the calorific mass.

The SAR assessment using temperature is less used than the method based on the electric field. In addition to sensitivity, another problem of the SAR measurement via the temperature is linked to the need of a steady state before each measurement. In case of a large number of measurement points, this constraint can induce long durations for the measurement, which is not always compatible with other constraints such as the life of wireless phone batteries. Because of this, the compliance of mobile phones is performed through the electric field assessment.

Eectric field measurement using small antennas, detection sensors or optical probes is nowadays the most common method used to experimentally assess SAR. Equation [1.4], that will be explained in section 2.2.5.2, provides the relationship between the SAR and the electric field.

$$\mathrm{SAR} = \frac{\sigma E^2}{2\rho} \qquad [1.4]$$

where σ, ρ and E represent, respectively, the conductivity of the body tissue (S/m), the mass density of the tissue (kg/m^3) and the peak electric field strength in the tissue (V/m). Depending on the use of r ms (root mean square) or maximum value of the electric field strength, the coefficient ½ exists or not. In this book, coefficient ½ will be used.

1.2.2. *Protection limits*

1.2.2.1. *Basic restrictions*

To protect humans from the adverse health effects of EMFs, ICNIRP, IEEE and the International Committee on Electromagnetic Safety (ICES) have agreed on a set of recommended limits [ICN 98, IEE 05].

ICNIRP limits are composed of fundamental ones – the *basic restrictions* – and derived ones – the *reference levels.*

Basic restrictions are, on the one hand, the local exposure, and, on the other hand, the exposure averaged over the whole body, using SAR. These limits are established to protect humans from the known health effects.

In the RF domain, these are the thermal effects. As stated in the ICNIRP guidelines, with an exposure higher than 4 W/kg for longer than 6 min, the rise in human body temperature can be higher than 1°C, which can induce possibly adverse health effects.

To protect from such thermal effects, an exposure limitation of 0.4 W/kg has been recommended for a healthy adult (and, by extension, also defined for workers). The maximum recommended exposure is therefore 10 times below the level which includes a thermal effect. With regard to the general public, taking into account a possible specificity of young children, elderly or sick people, an additional safety factor of 5 has been also defined.

Ultimately, the whole body averaged SAR (WBSAR) limit for general public is 0.08 W/kg and for workers is 0.4 W/kg. A similar approach has been used to define local limits. Health effects have been reported with local exposure above 100 W/kg ICNIRP. Therefore, for head and trunk, a limit of 2 W/kg (50 times below the health effect) has been recommended for the general public and 10 W/kg (10 times below the health effect) for workers. For the limbs, the general public and worker limits are, respectively, 10 and 20 W/kg. All these limits are summarized in Table 1.1.

Basic restrictions	Public	Workers
Whole body SAR (W/kg)	0.08	0.4
Local SAR (W/kg) Head – Trunk	2	10
Local SAR (W/kg) Limbs	4	20

Table 1.1. *ICNIRP basic restrictions*

1.2.2.2. *From basic restrictions to reference levels*

The measurement of SAR is complex and requires a laboratory. *Reference levels* have been defined to help reinforce the *basic restrictions*. They define a limit for the incident field strength that is the level inducing an exposure compliant with the *basic restrictions*.

Since SAR assessment could not be performed *in situ* in the 1960s, studies were conducted to characterize a transfer function of the incident EMF to the power absorbed by the human body. The initial studies were carried out with analytical approaches and mathematical structures such as spheroids. This relationship was then revisited in the 2000s using advanced numerical methods and phantoms [WU 11, CON 08].

As an antenna, the "equivalent surface" of the body evolves with the frequency; as a consequence, while the basic restrictions do not depend on the frequency, the reference levels are frequency dependent.

Human morphology is variable and body shape, as well as internal organ proportions, can vary; because of this, as shown in Figure 1.2, the power absorbed by a human body depends on the frequency and morphology. Figure 1.2 also shows, for different human body models, in standing positions, the whole body SAR versus the frequency.

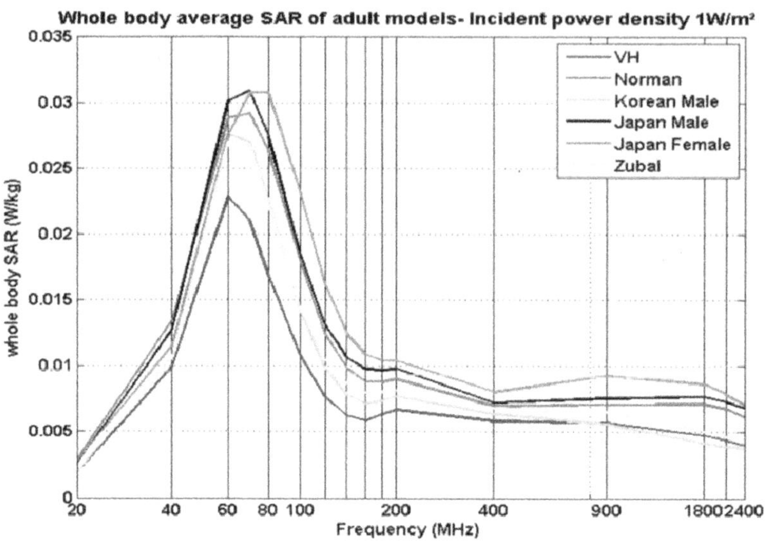

Figure 1.2. *Whole body averaged SAR for different body modelversus frequency. For a color version of the figure, see www.iste.co.uk/wiart/radiofrequency.zip*

From the EMF point of view, the "equivalent surface" of the body depends on the angle of incidence that is therefore also an important parameter [CON 11]. Figure 1.3 shows, with the Thelonius model [CHR 10], the whole body SAR variation due to the incidence angle (in the plane perpendicular to the vertical body).

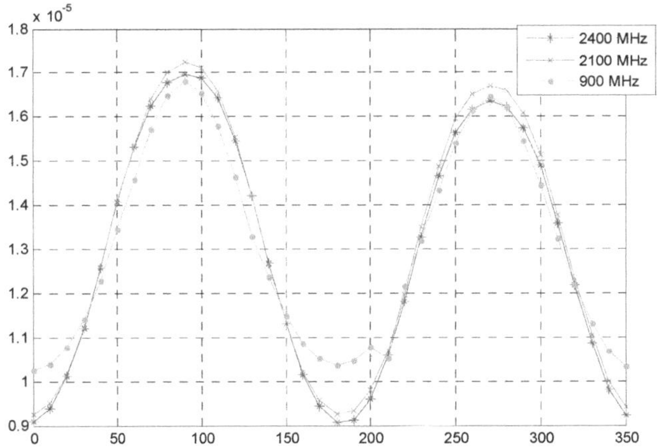

Figure 1.3. *Thelonius whole body SAR, in Watt/kg, versus angle of incidence for exposure. For a color version of the figure, see www.iste.co.uk/wiart/radiofrequency.zip*

To define the *reference levels*, studies analyzed the incident field strength that induces a whole body averaged SAR below 0.08 W/kg.

As described previously, the *reference levels* are frequency dependent and in the frequency band [60–100 MHz], the human body has a higher capability (from the equivalent surface point of view) to absorb electromagnetic energy. In this frequency band, the adult human body size (e.g. height between 1.5 and 1.8 m) is close to a quarter wave length. Because of that, the admissible maximum power density must be lower than elsewhere. Above 2 GHz, the human absorption is much more local and less dependent on the frequency. In this case, the admissible maximum power density is constant. Figure 1.2 also shows that this "resonance" depends on the morphology and posture. The smaller the body size, the higher the frequency at this resonance.

To define protection limits, the dependency of "resonance" on morphology has to be compatible with the human population (large people, small people, etc.). Based on these analyses and results, ICNIRP has defined the reference levels that are summarized in Table 1.2.

As explained previously, the basic restrictions do not depend on frequency but as Figure 1.2 shows, the transfer function from incident field to the whole body absorption depends on the frequency. A multi-source or multi-frequency exposure analysis with the reference levels therefore requires special attention.

Frequency range	E-field strength (V.m^{-1})	H-field strength (A.m^{-1})	B-field (μT)	Equivalent plane wave power density S_{eq} (W.m^{-2})
up to 1 Hz	–	3.2×10^4	4×10^4	–
1–8 Hz	10,000	$3.2 \times 10^4/f^2$	$4 \times 10^4/f^2$	–
8–25 Hz	10,000	$4{,}000/f$	$5{,}000/f$	–
0.025–0.8 Hz	$250/f$	$4/f$	$5/f$	–
0.8–3 Hz	$250/f$	5	6.25	–
3–150 Hz	87	5	6.25	–
0.15–1 Hz	87	$0.73/f$	$0.92/f$	–
1–10 Hz	$87/f^{1/2}$	$0.73/f$	$0.92/f$	–
10–400 Hz	28	0.073	0.092	2
400–2000 Hz	$1.375/f^{1/2}$	$0.0037/f^{1/2}$	$0.0046/f^{1/2}$	$f/200$
2–300 Hz	61	0.16	0.20	10

Note

1. f as indicated in the frequency range column.

2. Provided that basic restrictions are met and adverse indirect effects can be excluded, field strength values can be exceeded.

3. For frequencies between 100 kHz and 10 GHz, Seq, E2, H2, and B2 are to averaged over any 6-min period.

4.Between 100 kHz and 10 MHz, peak values for the field strengths are obtained by interpolation from the 1.5-fold peak at 100 kHz to the 32-fold peak at 10 MHz. For frequencies exceeding 10 MHz it is suggested that the peak equivalent plane wave power density, as averaged over the pulse width does not exceed 1,000times the Seq restrictions, or that the field strength does not exceed 32 times the field strength exposure levels given in the table.

5.For frequencies exceeding 10 GHz, Seq, E2, H2, and B2 are to be averaged over any 68/f 1.05-min period (f in GHz).

Table 1.2. *ICNIRP reference levels for general public (from [ICN 98])*

Let us consider two sources of exposure, S_1 and S_2, with their different frequencies, f_1 and f_2, and their EMF strengths, $\{E_1, H_1\}\{E_2, H_2\}$. In such a configuration, even if the incident field strength is the same, the whole body absorption, occurring at frequency f_1, can be different from that at frequency f_2. Let us also consider the references levels, L_1 and L_2, linked, respectively, to the frequencies f_1 and f_2. The EMF supporting the information coming from these sources can be expressed as a function of frequency, f_i, phase, $\phi_i(x, y, z, t)$, location $\{x, y, z\}$ and time t, for instance, and assuming a sine function and a time delay T_i (delay due to the propagation), the electric field in time domain is given by [1.5]:

$$E_i = E_i\sqrt{2}\sin\left[2\pi f_i(t - T_i) + \phi_i(t) + 2\pi f_i T_i\right] \quad [1.5]$$

The time averaging of E_i (denoted as $< E_i >$) will provide the field strength of the field that can be used to assess the exposure.

If we assume, on the one hand, $L_1 = L_2 = L$ in the frequency bands of the signals emitted by S_1 and S_2, and on the other hand, the non-coherence of the phases, $\phi_i(t)$, of these signals, then the total exposure induced by the sources S_1 and S_2 is given by the root mean square of the component and the incident field strength is given by [1.6]:

$$E = \sqrt{E_1{}^2 + E_2{}^2} \qquad [1.6]$$

If we assume now that $L_1 \neq L_2$, then the exposure cannot be managed as it was before. In such a configuration, as shown in Figure 1.2, even if the incident field strength is the same, the whole body absorption at f_1 can be different from that at f_2. In this case, the quantity given by $\sqrt{E_1{}^2 + E_2{}^2}$ cannot be used to check the compliance to the limit. In such a configuration, the objective is to verify that the sum of the percentages of the relative limits is less than 100%. Let us consider the limits L_1 and L_2 at frequencies f_1 and f_2. According to previous sections, the source S_1 and S_2 are, respectively, inducing $\left(\frac{E_1}{L_1}\right)^2$ and $\left(\frac{E_2}{L_2}\right)^2$ percent of their respective limits.

To be compliant with the ICNIRP limits, the exposure induced by E_1 and E_2 must comply with [1.7]

$$\left[\left(\frac{E_1}{L_1}\right)^2 + \left(\frac{E_2}{L_2}\right)^2\right] \leq 1 \qquad [1.7]$$

The general public often considers such an approach as being complex. To help with the comparisons, some countries for example France, have introduced a new metric: "xx V/m equivalent f MHz". To be comparable to E_1 emitted at f_1, the field E_2 emitted at f_2 has to be weighed by a coefficient $\sqrt{\left(\frac{L_1}{L_2}\right)}$. Using this approach, 6 V/m at 2 GHz is equal to 4 V/m "equivalent 900 MHz".

If the sources are emitting at the same frequency and if the phases are coherent, as we have with multiple reflections and narrow band signals, the interferences, inside the human body, exist and must be taken into account. The studies that have been carried out with narrow band signals (e.g. GSM) [VER 10, KIE 11] show variations. Figure 1.4 shows the variation of the "Thelonius" exposure induced by five incident plane waves having vertical polarization. In this case, the amplitude and the phase follow, respectively, a log-normal and a uniform distribution and the total exposure is normalized ($\sum_1^5 {E_i}^2 = 1$). The ratio of the standard deviation to the mean value of the whole body SAR is 25%.

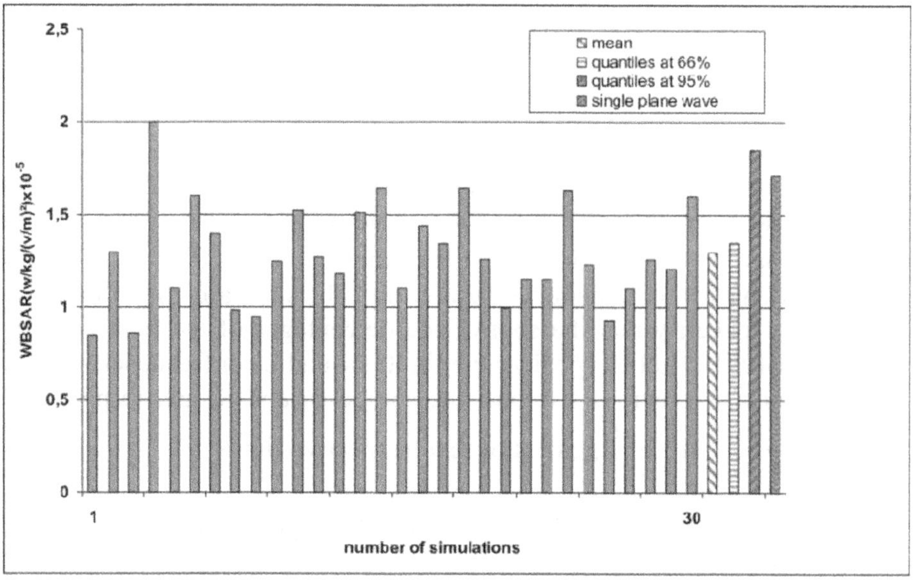

Figure 1.4. *Thelonius whole body SAR versus angle of incidence for exposure induced by five incident plane waves having vertical polarization, log-normal distribution for the amplitude and uniform distribution for the phase. For a color version of the figure, see www.iste.co.uk/wiart/radiofrequency.zip*

1.2.3. *Exposure assessment for compliance tests*

1.2.3.1. *Introduction*

The methods and protocols that have been analyzed and specified for compliance tests can be shared in three large domains linked to tests dedicated to:

– put mobile phones on the market;

– putting radio base stations (RBSs) on the market;

– putting the RBSs into service.

For the methods and protocols that have been dedicated to mobiles, most of the works carried out have been dedicated to defining methods and protocols applicable in specialized laboratories. The primary objective of these works was first to define a standardized head phantom, second to define a homogeneous liquid (the "equivalent head tissues") to fill the head phantom and lastly to standardize the tests positions (relatively to the head) of the equipment under test (EUT). The phantom, liquid and positions are designed in such a way that the SAR assessed using these standardized head, liquid and test positions will never exceed the maximum SAR that can be induced by the EUT in a real head.

The first step has been to develop and agree on the phantom head shape and on the equivalent liquid. The studies that have been conducted to develop a phantom shape have led to the well-known "SAM" (Specific Anthropomorphic Mannequin) head, now used in CENELEC, IEC and IEEE standards.

The "head equivalent" liquid has been studied using multi-layers [DRO 00] and a heterogeneous head [MON 03]. Worldwide efforts have been conducted on this topic; comparisons of SAR in the SAM phantom to that in anatomically correct head models were also conducted [BEA 06] using different types of incident fields and mobile phone models. In France, most of these studies were conducted in the framework of the COMOBIO RNRT research program [GRA 03].

The *E* field measurement in the phantom and the estimation of the averaged SAR more than 10 g is based on sampling measurements performed with a robot. Studies were carried out to develop efficient interpolation methods applicable to SAR [BRI 08, BRI 01].

The first standards were dedicated to mobile phones close to the head since this usage was the quasi-unique way to use a handset. Wireless communication usages have evolved. With hand-free kit or speaker mode, and with the development of connected objects located close to the body, the compliance tests have also evolved. Tests performed with EUT close to the head were not enough. New standards were developed to specify tests to conduct for products that can be used close to the body. A new flat phantom able to represent the body was defined and a new equivalent liquid was studied. The equivalent liquid used in the standards dedicated to mobiles was initially based on head tissues; they are obviously not the same as in other parts of the body. International studies were performed to check in which conditions the equivalent head liquid can be used for SAR assessment of EUT close to the body. In particular, the studies analyzed possible correction factors [PRA 08] that can be used to correct measurements performed in the flat phantom using the equivalent head tissues.

The second domain is linked to the methods and protocols that have been dedicated to "put radio base stations on the market". These methods do not take into account the existing sources of EMF that exist when the product will be put into service, at a given location. The methods and protocols that have been studied for putting devices on the market are mainly in lab tests or based on antenna numerical modeling. Their objectives are to specify methods which verify the compliance to the basic restriction or to the reference levels, and, if needed, specify the compliance boundaries that guaranty an exposure below the limit outside these areas. These methods have been developed taking into account the large research efforts carried out for the standard dedicated to the mobile. Despite these efforts, the use of reference levels is easier than complex SAR assessments. Works have therefore been conducted to define efficient methods to verify compliance to the reference levels.

With the power emitted by cellular telecommunication RBSs, the compliance distances, also known as "safety perimeter" compliance boundaries, are not often in the far field of the antenna. For instance, with a typical base station array antenna, composed of eight dipoles and length of 2 m, the "far field" distance is larger than 10 m. Because of this, the easy-to-use, far field gain formulas cannot be used since they are not valid in the near field. To overcome this problem, efforts have been dedicated to developing, in the near field of the antennas, efficient models for base station antennas (BSAs) usable for human exposure assessment [ALT 08, FA 00].

Sub-antenna modeling [ALT 08] has been developed to respond to this demand. This approach is based on the superposition principle and is suitable for most broadcast and cellular antennas based on collinear arrays.

In this case, as shown in Figure 1.5, the antenna can be seen as a sum of basic elements. If the coupling between sub-elements is negligible, then the total *E* field is the sum (vector) of the *E* field induced by the sub-elements.

$$\vec{\mathrm{E}} = \sum_i \beta_i \vec{\mathrm{E}}_i(r_i, \theta_i, \varphi_i) \qquad [1.8]$$

The main advantage of this approach is to be able to use a far field formula of the sub-element in the near field of the total antenna.

In this model, we can consider the coefficient β_i as independent of the sub-antenna. In this case, this coefficient can be determined using the array factor and the power delivered to the antenna. In fact, the collinear array antennas are often designed to reduce the energy spent in side mode. Because of that, the sub-antenna alimentation (amplitude and phase) is not uniform and depends on the tilt and side lobes of the total antenna.

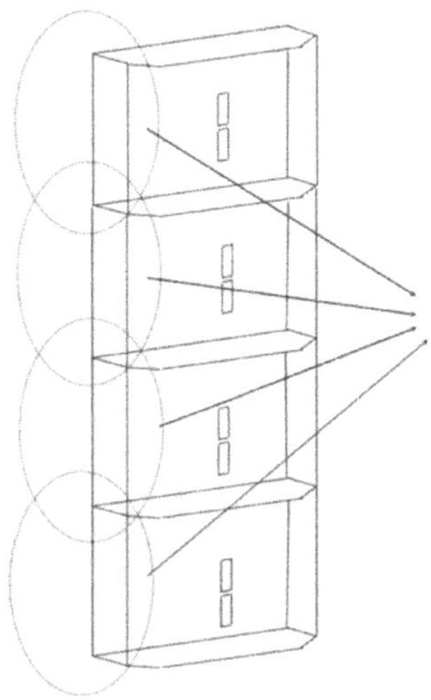

Figure 1.5. *Antenna modeling using sub-antenna approach*

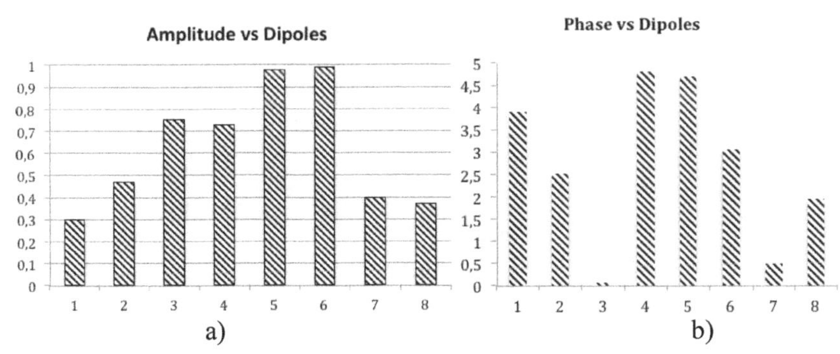

Figure 1.6. *Example of amplitude a) and phase b) applied to the eight dipoles of an array antenna*

The E field in the far field can be used to determine the pattern of alimentation achieving the far field gain pattern. Spherical modes, genetic algorithms and a cost function based on the maxima of the far field gain can also be used [ADA 04] to determine the amplitude and phase (see Figure 1.6) that can be used to model efficiency base station for human exposure. Figure 1.7 shows the electric field assessed using spherical modes and sub-antenna.

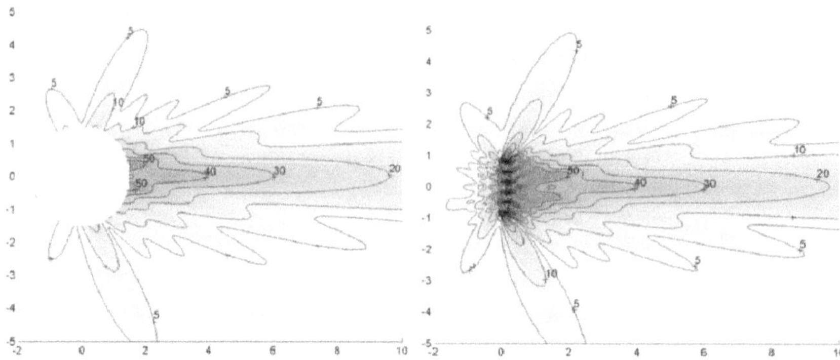

Figure 1.7. *E field obtained through spherical modes a) and sub-antenna modeling b)*

Such models are nowadays used in the commercial software EMF-Visual (www.satimo.fr). Figure 1.8 shows an example of visual use for compliance boundary and field strength prediction based on sub-antenna modeling.

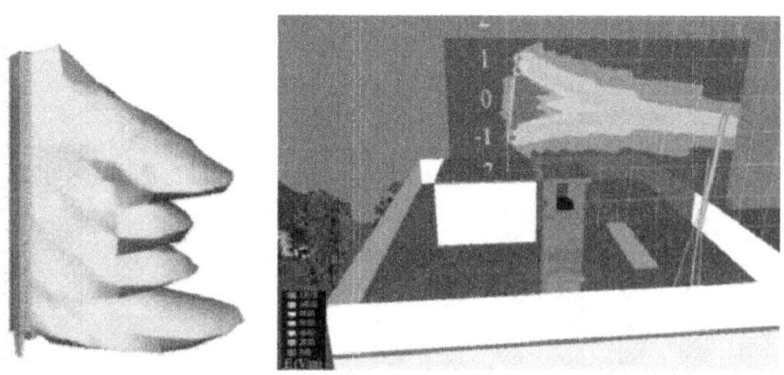

Figure 1.8. *EMF visual use (compliance boundary a), field b) of sub-antenna models. For a color version of the figure, see www.iste.co.uk/wiart/radiofrequency.zip*

The reference levels are necessary to guarantee compliance to basic restrictions. Because of this, the compliance distance is often larger than that obtained using SAR assessment. When the antenna of the wireless devices are close to the body, the coupling between the antennas and body exist and the SAR measurement must be used to check the compliance to limits.

Because of this, flat phantom specifications have been developed by CENELEC and IEC to test small antenna. To simplify the procedures, studies were conducted on possible correction factors to be used [PRA 08] when the equivalent head liquid, recommended in the standard dedicated to mobiles, is used for other parts of the body.

The use of reference levels to define boundary limits can lead to obtaining a large area, compared to what is really needed if the basic restrictions are used for a specific product. Plane wave decomposition and simplified formulas for the exposure to radio base station antennas have been studied to optimize the boundary limits [GOS 11, SAI 08, NIC 04].

Important works have also been carried out to specify methods that can be used to put base stations "into service". In this case, studies have been carried out to characterize and quantify, on the one hand, the influence of the emission of the antenna put into service on the existing compliance boundary (linked to other sources) and, on the other hand, the influence of EMF induced by existing sources on the compliance boundary defined in the lab and in the absence of these pre-existing sources.

1.2.3.2. *SAR assessment for compliance test*

Depending on the technology, the power emitted by devices can be highly variable and depends on protocol and network technologies such as adaptive power control and handover [WIA 00, GAT 09]. The tests that have to be conducted, prior to putting devices on the market or into service, must take this variability into account. It is therefore fundamental to establish sound methods and design measurement systems able to guaranty that the devices are safe in all realistic configurations.

The main advantage of the measurement is the capability to assess the field and the SAR induced by an existing device, avoiding uncertainty linked to the modeling, but the main limitation is linked to the invasive approach. On the one hand, the SAR in the brain, for instance, cannot be performed on living individuals. On the other hand, the SAR assessment is complex in heterogeneous tissues, because of the modification in the tissue distribution in the vicinity of the sensor. It can be bypassed using “worst-case” scenarios; for instance, using a large phantom head (SAM) with an equivalent head liquid designed to overestimate the exposure, as they are in the compliance tests.

In line with this context, large international efforts have been performed over the last decades. In France, national research projects *Comobio*, *Adonis*, *Merodas* and *Multipass*, granted by ANR (*Agence Nationale de la Recherche*), have investigated the basic requirements for measurement equipment and measurement protocols to assess the human exposure and design experimental systems (e.g. Figure 1.9), allowing for SAR assessment. Based on these international works, carried out in the 1990s, the compliance tests and basic requirement applicable to usage close to the head have been standardized and described in technical standards.

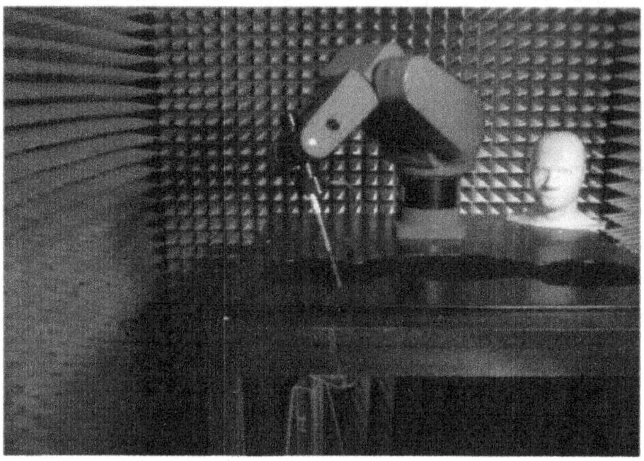

Figure 1.9. *SAR measurement system*

A large part of the studies carried out was dedicated to the probes, the *E* field scanning system [POK 00, CHE 96, GRA 03] and the dielectric properties of human tissues [GAB 96a, GAB 96b, GAB 96c]. Several other studies have been analyzed, using numerical simulations, the equivalent tissues, test positions and SAM phantom shape to guaranty that the SAR induced by a device in a real head will be always below the SAR measurement performed in the SAM phantom.

Numerical methods such as the finite difference in time domain (FDTD) or multilayer approaches have been used to determine the properties of the tissues equivalent liquid that fills the phantom [DRO 00, MON 03]. The dielectric properties of this liquid have not been defined as a simple averaging of the dielectric properties of human tissues. The liquid has been designed to handle a different morphology and guaranty a conservative assessment of the SAR (i.e. the SAR induced by a device in a real head will always be below the SAR assessed in the phantom SAM).

With the evolving usage of telecommunication networks, wireless devices are not only used close to the head but also close to the body (e.g. talk mode, streaming, etc.). Studies have therefore been performed to define new equivalent liquids that can be used with RF sources close to some parts of the body other than the head [PRA 08].

One of the very practical problems encountered during the design of the compliance tests was linked to the limited lifetime of the mobile's battery allowing, among other things, the emission of this latter. Indeed, during compliance tests, a mobile phone will use its own battery. Because of this, the SAR measurement of a device has to be performed within a limited time and so with a limited number of measurements. To overcome these limits, interpolation and extrapolation schemes [BRI 08, BRI 01] have been analyzed. The positions ("cheek" and "tilt") of the EUT relative to the head have been standardized (Figure 1.10) as well as the shape of the phantom and the equivalent liquid [GRA 03, WIA 01, BEA 06].

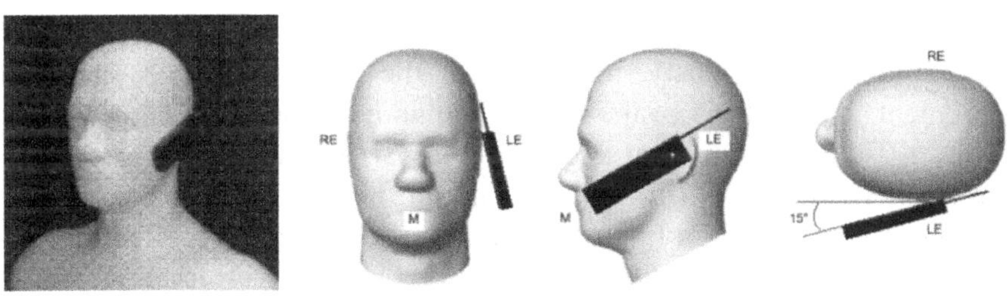

Figure 1.10. *SAM phantom and test positions*

The power emitted by wireless communication systems is not necessarily constant. As shown in Figure 1.11, and as was pointed out at the beginning of this section, the power emitted by a cellular mobile is highly variable. To guarantee a conservative approach of the SAR assessment, the tests performed to check the compliance of EUT are, in line with the standards, performed with the maximum emitted power (in this case, the exposure is maximum).

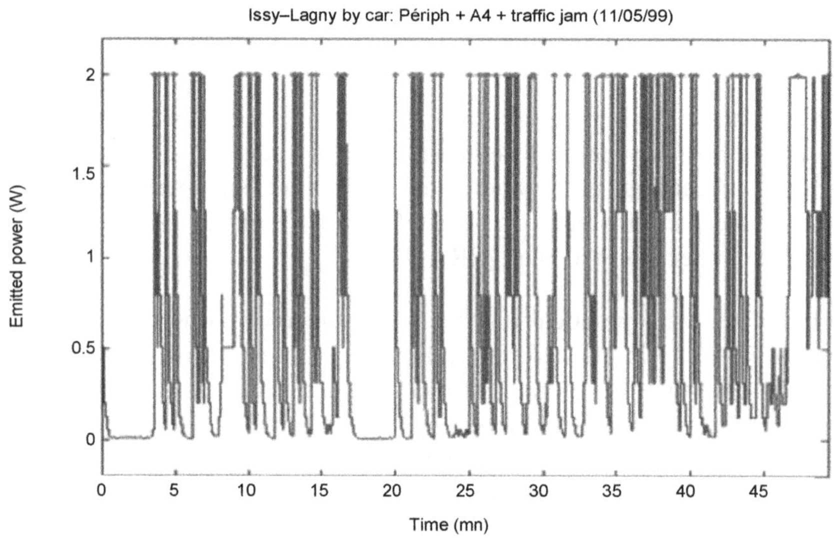

Figure 1.11. *Influence of the adaptive power control on the power transmitted by a GSM phone in an operating network*

1.2.3.3. *Field measurements for compliance tests*

As explained previously, because of the complexity of the SAR measurement, the analysis of the *in situ* human exposure is often performed using the E field measurement and with comparisons to "reference levels". In complex environments (in particular urban ones), the field received at a given point results in possibly a combination of obstructions, reflections and diffractions [WIA 95, ROS 00]; the variations induced by the environment on the received signal (see Figure 1.12) are often decomposed into "shadowing" and "fast fading".

"Shadowing" is mainly linked to environmental obstructions (e.g. a building) that affect the propagation of the energy. The variations linked to shadowing exist, as shown in Figure 1.12, over quite a large distance.

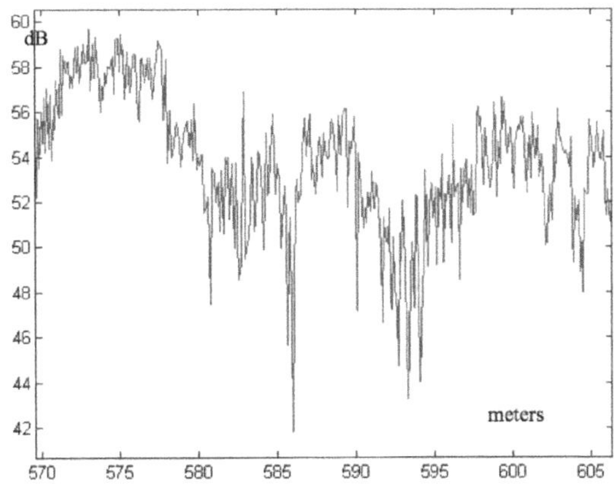

Figure 1.12. *Observed received signal variations induced by the environment*

Conversely, "fast fading" is a phenomenon affecting the incident field locally. Because of reflections and diffractions, depending on the environment complexity and the bandwidth of the signal, interferences can exist and produce local variations. They are known as "fast fading" (see Figure 1.13) and affect the field strength.

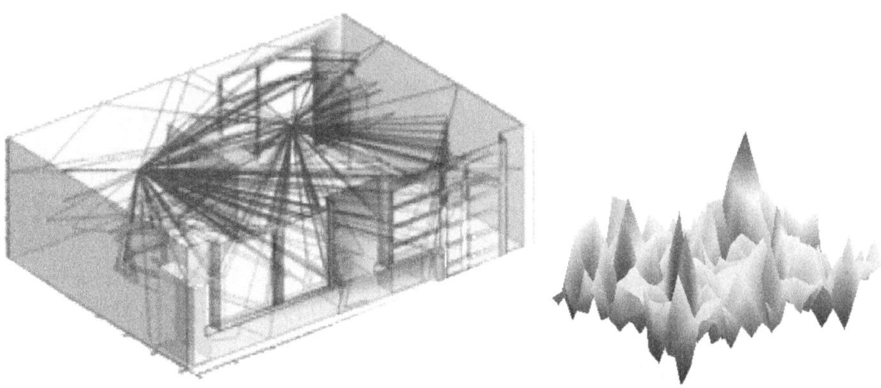

Figure 1.13. *Multipath exposure induced by a source in indoor (left) and local E field strength spatial distribution (right). For a color version of the figure, see www.iste.co.uk/wiart/radiofrequency.zip*

Because of this, a narrow band measurement performed at a given location can vary from a measurement performed 50 cm away. It is therefore important to define a robust method to assess the human exposure at a given location.

Because of the possible fast fading, exposure assessment is often not possible with measurements performed at only one point. CENELEC EN 50492 and IEC-62232 have defined a protocol to estimate the incident field over the human cross-section. Different averaging methods, such as those shown in Figure 1.14, are proposed in the standards. The key question is to estimate the uncertainty of the estimation.

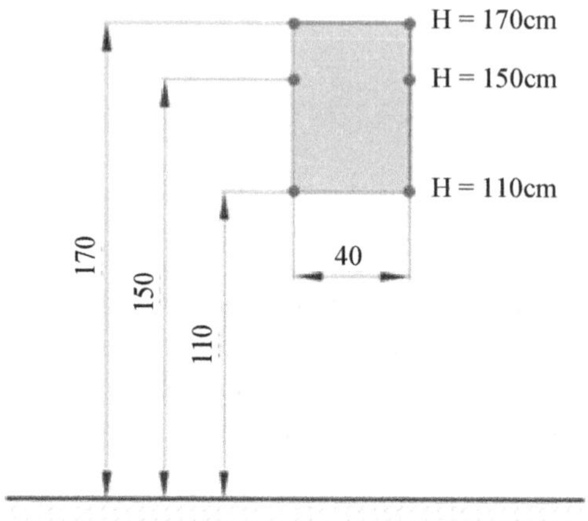

Figure 1.14. *Example of location of measurement points for spatial averaging*

Depending on the environment, local variations of the E field strength can follow different statistical laws and have an influence on the accuracy of the mean assessment. Studies have been performed [LAR 05] to estimate the uncertainty at 95% on the power density exposure (see Figure 1.15) and have been used in standards such as CENELEC EN 50492 and IEC 62232.

The traffic supported by cellular networks can influence the power emitted by the RSB. Figure 1.16 shows such variations in case of a GSM base station emitting at 1,800 MHz. To guarantee compliance to legal limits, as explained previously, worst cases are often used. The objective is, in this case, to assess a reliable radiated field value considering all the surrounding

BSAs emitting at their maximum power as they are expected to work in a full traffic situation.

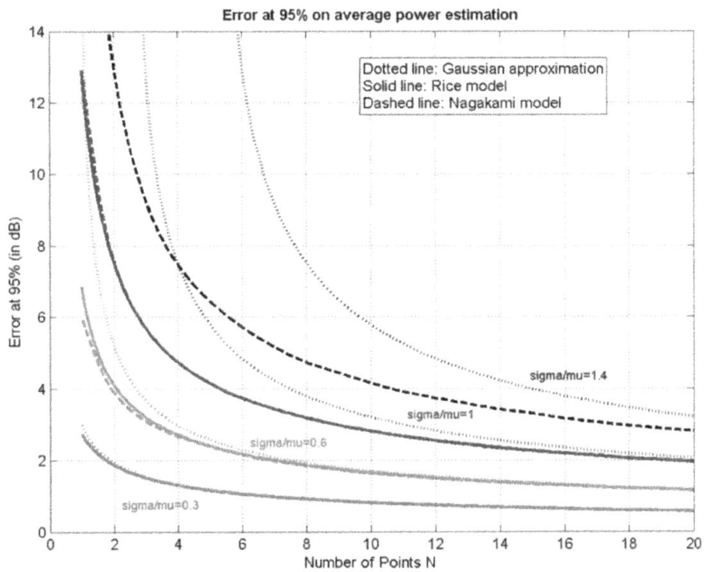

Figure 1.15. *Error at 95% of the incident power estimation versus the number of points. For a color version of the figure, see www.iste.co.uk/wiart/radiofrequency.zip*

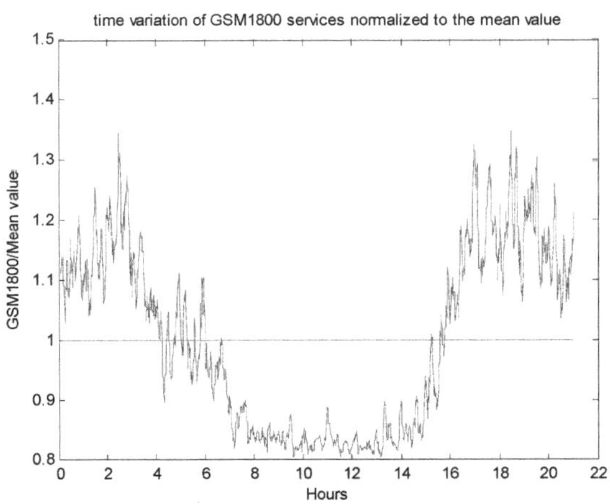

Figure 1.16. *Time variation of the field emitted, normalized to the mean value, by a GSM base station antenna emitting at 1,800 MHz*

Cellular networks are evolving. In Europe, most networks were “2G” (GSM) in the 1990s, then “3G” (UMTS) appeared in the 2000s and “4G” (LTE) in the 2010s. “5G” is being developed and should be commercialized in 2020. These networks do not use the same protocol and radio access technology (RAT): “2G” is based on time division multiple access, “3G” on code division multiple access and “4G” on orthogonal frequency-division multiplexing (OFDM). The strategy to estimate the maximum exposure has to take into account the specificity of the technologies and networks. For instance, a GSM downlink signal is composed of a constant power signal named the BCCH (broadcast common channel) and several other channels (TRX) used for transporting the connected users communications. BCCH and TRX use different frequency bands. The BCCH carrier can also be used for transporting communication, however, its power is not affected by any power control and is maintained constant using “padding bits”. The worst-case situation, at a given location, induced by one base station, can be based on the measurement, at this location, of the signal associated to the BCCH multiply by the number of transmitters. While GSM is based on TDMA, the UMTS signal is based on WCDMA technique. All the users connected to the BS antenna share at the same time the same bandwidth of 5 MHz. The equivalent in “3G” of the previous BCCH used in “2G” is the common pilot channel (CPICH). In 3G, the number of TRX is the proportion of common channel power to the maximum power delivered by the antenna. As for the GSM, the first parameter can be measured and the second is set up by the operator and should be considered as close to 10% (3 GPP guidelines).

1.2.4. *Real exposure assessment*

1.2.4.1. *Exposure induced by access points*

Worst-cases are often used to guarantee the compliance of exposure levels to legal limits. As a consequence, the tests are carried out to check, using a conservative extrapolation (see previous section), the compliance of the EMF exposure induced by base stations (down link) to the relevant limits.

As an example, the exposure induced by GSM BSA can be overestimated using the measurement of the BCCH (the broadcast common channel that is always emitting and not affected by power control) multiplied by the number of transmitters (TRX) linked to the BCCH channel. In such a case, if at a given location $E_{\max}$ is the electric field induced by the BCCH and n_{trx} the number of relative TRX, then at maximum traffic the maximum exposure can be overestimated by [1.9]:

$$E_{\max} = E_{\text{bcch}}\sqrt{n_{\text{trx}}} \qquad [1.9]$$

The overestimation method can be extrapolated to other technology such as 3G where the relevant stable quantity is not the BCCH, that does not exist, but the CPITCH [BSI 08]. Such an approach is fundamental but not always sufficient to inform the general public and assess the real exposure induced by different networks.

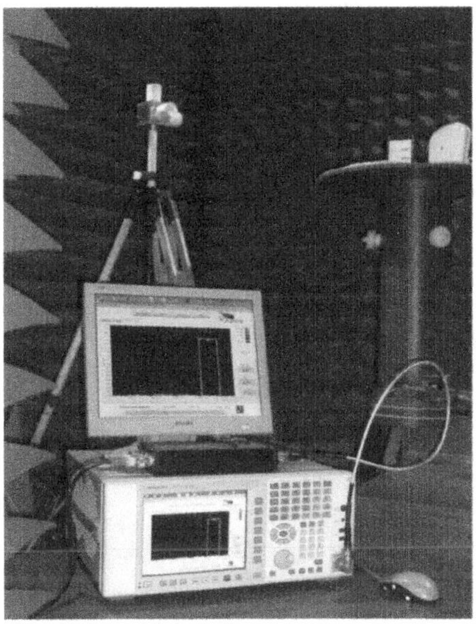

Figure 1.17. *Spectrum measurement "Xplora" composed of a three-axis antenna and a spectrum analyzer*

Several projects, such as the ANR *Multipass* project in France, have been setup to characterize the real exposure induced by communication networks. Using specific equipment (Figure 1.17) composed of a three-axis probe and spectrum analyzer, E field measurements have been carried over duration of 24 h and longer with a sampling of few seconds (Figure 1.18).

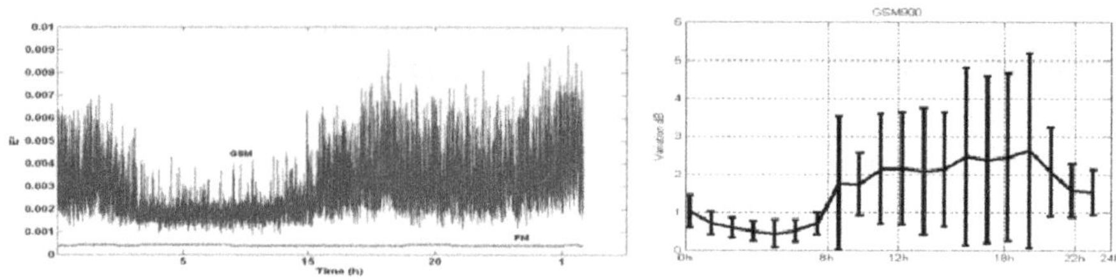

Figure 1.18. *E field measurement over 24h for the E field induced by a GSM base station operating at 900 MHz and FM (left). Variation of the power density of the GSM signal (right)*

As shown in Figure 1.18, with GSM technology, the E field varies because of the traffic variations but is well below the theoretical maximum. The traffic variations and pattern of use depend on the technology, but whatever the technology, operating networks are designed to avoid saturation. Because of this, the maximum theoretical exposure (i.e. all the channel emitting at maximum) is below the maximum maximorum. The real extrapolation factor is therefore below the theoretical factor. Measurements of the real extrapolation factor have been performed and analyzed in various environments [MAH 11, MAH 12]. As shown in Figure 1.19, the cumulative distribution function (CDF) of the extrapolation factor linked to GSM 900, GSM 1800, UMTS and HSPA is a worst-case inducing a strong overestimation of the real exposure; for instance, in 99% of the cases the extrapolation factor is less than 2 while in theory it can be up to 10.

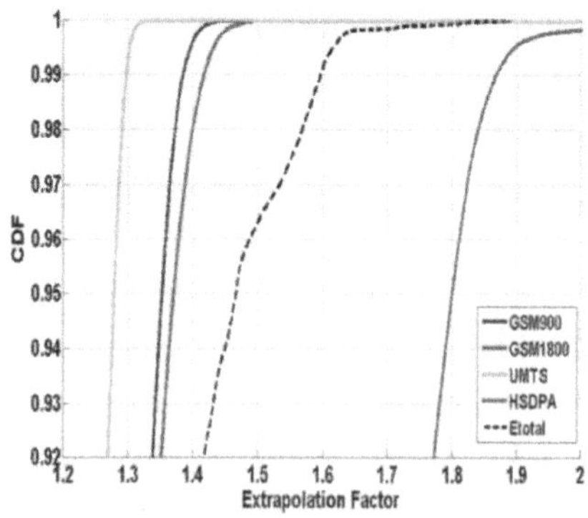

Figure 1.19. *CDF real ratio between the real exposure and the BCCH. For a color version of the figure, see www.iste.co.uk/wiart/radiofrequency.zip*

1.2.4.2. *Real exposure induced by devices*

1.2.4.2.1. Emitted power in voice circuit mode

In voice circuit mode, the bandwidth of the signal is constant and the signal-to-noise ratio (SNR) achieved at the radio BSA location depends mainly on the power received at the BSA. A target SNR is required to have a good communication quality. Because of the environment and because of the movement of the user, the power emitted by the device has to be modified to have an SNR close to the target one at the BSA location. As shown in Figure 1.20, the power emitted by devices is highly variable and depends on the protocols used and network technologies. This is due to the adaptive power control strategy but also because of the handover management that depends on the network technologies.

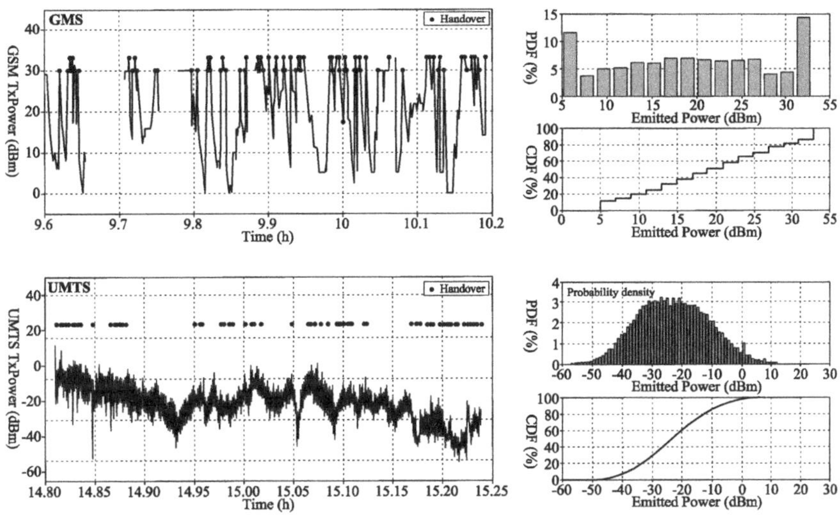

Figure 1.20. *Example of power emitted by GSM and UMTS devices in operational networks and in voice circuit modes*

1.2.4.2.2. Emitted power in data mode

In voice circuit mode, the data rate requested is known and constant; conversely, in data mode, the data rate depends on the capability of the network and on the network's management of the resources. Let us consider a speech of 60 s, it will be encoded in a file of 1,800 kb (with an usual encoder of 30 kb/s of speech). This file can be transmitted in less than 6 s with technologies such as 3G and 4G that have the uplink transmitted data rate higher than 300 kb/s. According to Shannon [SHA 49], in the presence of noise, the maximum rate at which data can be transmitted over a communication channel of a specified bandwidth depends on the energy per byte received by the receiver. This energy per byte depends on the environment (attenuation, diffraction, distance) and on the power emitted by the transmitter. The noise also depends on the information transmitted by other devices in the communication channel. Because of that, in data mode, the duration of the data transmission, the data rate, the resources management, the power emitted and the network load can be highly correlated.

This is important for epidemiological studies. With the voice circuit, the mean human exposure can be linked to the mean power emitted during the call duration. In data mode this is no longer valid: the call duration does not provide the real duration (in case of VoIP for instance) of the transmission.

Figure 1.21 shows with 3G the time variation in data mode of the transmitted power and the uplink data rate.

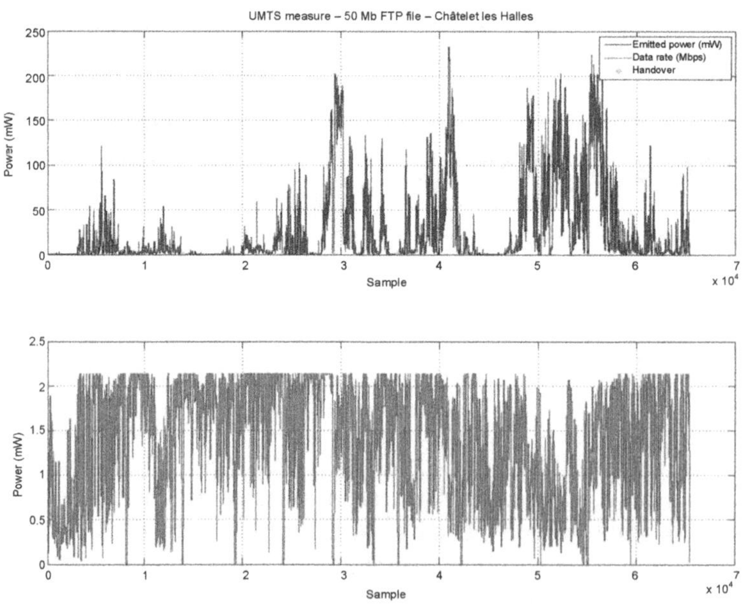

Figure 1.21. *Transmitted power and data rate versus time*

1.2.4.3. *Comparative analysis of the exposure induced by mobile phones and base stations*

As previously described, considerable efforts were conducted in the 1990s to draft product and basic standards dedicated to the compliance tests of wireless systems emitting EMF. Programs dedicated to monitor the EMF exposure of population have been set up in various countries, but most of these projects do not consider the global exposure induced by mobile and base stations. They consider them separately and focus on their compliance to the relevant limit. Current standards do not consider that the real EMF exposure is induced by both the "uplink" (the transmitted power (TX)) and the "downlink" (the received power (RX)), that are, as shown in Figure 1.22, highly correlated.

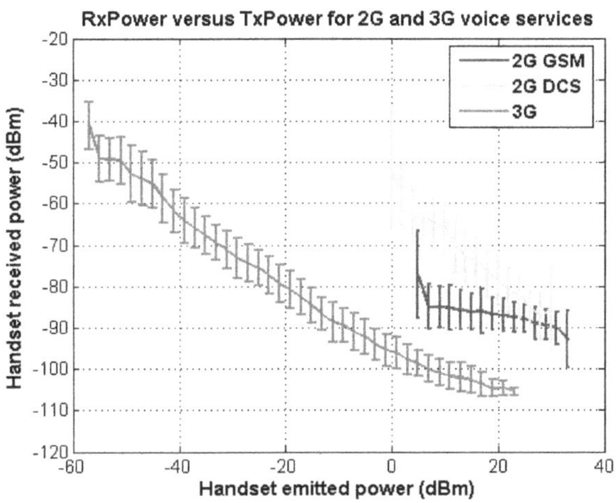

Figure 1.22. *Correlation between TX and RX for 2G and 3G services. For a color version of the figure, see www.iste.co.uk/wiart/radiofrequency.zip*

Since epidemiological studies are requesting the real exposure and not only the maximum one, several studies have been performed to estimate the real power emitted by mobile phones. Some of these studies [VRI 09, WRI 09, KEL 11] performed with systems such as test mobile phones (TEMS) or software-modified phones (SMP) have shown that handover management greatly influences the mean power emitted by GSM phones. Indeed, due to the GSM protocol, at each handover, the emitted power of wireless phones is set at the maximum authorized in the network cell, that is usually well above the needed power from the SNR point of view. After the handover, the power emitted decreases to reach the target SNR and avoid additional noise. As shown in the literature [VRI 09], in the 2000s and because of the handover management, the power emitted by GMS phone was often the maximum that could be emitted from phones. Because of this, the mean power emitted by GSM devices was about 50% of the maximum power.

Similar studies have been performed for UMTS phones [GAT 09]. The code division multiplex access (CDMA) used by UMTS is very sensitive to noise. Because of that, the UMTS handover management differs from the GSM one. With UMTS, the device is connected to several Radio Base Station Antenna (RBSA) (also known as "NODE B") and the power emitted by the phone is not affected by the handovers. The studies performed have shown that the median and mean power emitted by UMTS, in voice call usage, were, respectively, close to 0.1% and 1% of the maximum since the handover with UMTS does not induce a rise in power.

Figures 1.22 and 1.23 show the normalized mean power emitted (dB) and the power received (dBm) by mobiles used in a real cellular wireless communication network. The data were collected with special phones, like trace mobiles, but also using probes in the Orange network. These probes, which are in fact software, have grasped the information exchanged between devices and network.

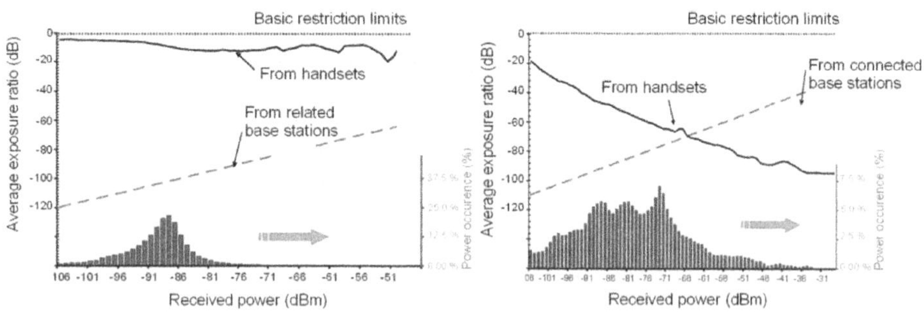

Figure 1.23. *TX (dB) versus RX (dBm) for 2G (left) and 3G (right) services*

With 3G networks, we can observe that the closer the devices are to the 3G base stations, the higher the power received and the lower the power emitted by these devices. We can also observe that in 2G, the power emitted decreases much less than in 3G, with the distance to base stations. This is due to, on the one hand, the power emitted by 2G devices that cannot be as low as in 3G, but, on the other hand, is also due to the handovers as explained previously.

Since in Europe people often complain about base stations, measurement protocols have been established to assess the exposure induced by RF system access points. In Europe, CENELEC TC106x has drafted and adopted a standard, EN50492, to measure the EMFs *in situ*. Studies have also been conducted in different countries to monitor the exposure induced by base stations [VIE 09, GAJ 13, TRO 08, JOS 12, BRE 09]. These measurements have shown that the exposure induced by base stations is weak (close to 0.1 V/m).

To compare the exposure induced by a mobile to those linked to the far field of the base station emission, the whole body SAR, as well as local SAR (e.g. maximum averaged SAR over 10 g), induced by a mobile phone and the SAR induced by base stations have been compared using simulations. The FDTD (see Chapter 2) has been used with a generic phone model [EUC 11], designed to induce 1 W/kg in SAM, and an environmental electric field, having a far field structure and a field strength E = 0.1 V/m. The SAR was calculated within two numerical human body models, "Duke" and "Thelonius" (see section 2.3.2) in "voice" and "data" postures as shown in Figure 1.24.

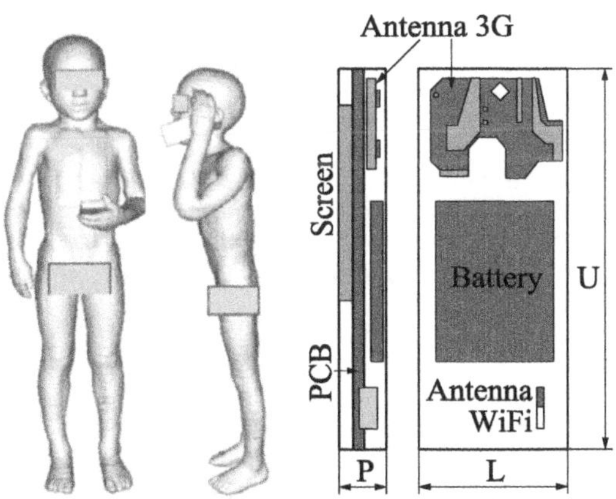

Figure 1.24. *"Thelonius" model in "data" (left) and "voice" (middle) configurations and a numerical phone model (right)*

The WBSAR, the maximum averaged SAR over 10 g in the head (max 10 g SAR) and the maximum averaged SAR over 1g in the brain (max 1 g brain) have been assessed for different frequencies (GSM and UMTS), postures (voice and data) and sources (phone model and plane wave as "far field"). The ratio of these quantities is summarized in Figure 1.25. Figure 1.25 shows that the exposure, whole body SAR and local SAR, induced by the mobile is, in the studied configurations, always higher than the same quantities induced by the base station. Figure 1.25 also shows that the ratio of the exposure induced by mobiles to those induced by base stations is higher with GSM than with UMTS. This is mainly due to the different power emitted (see section 1.2.4.2) but also due to the different frequency and spatial distribution of the power absorbed in the body.

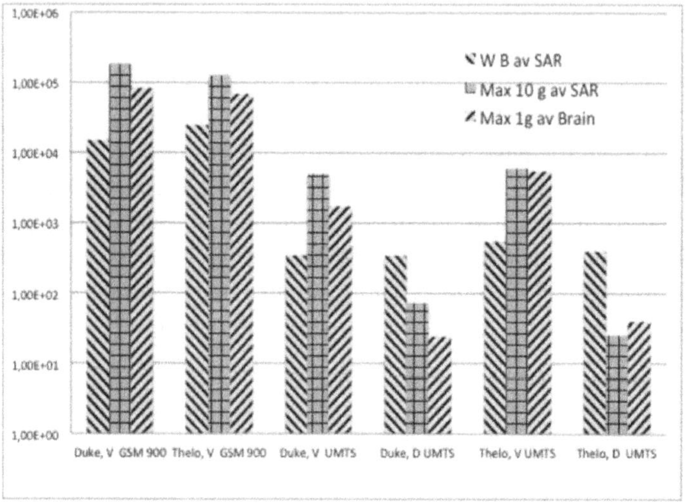

Figure 1.25. *Ratios of the whole body averaged SAR, max SAR averaged over 10 g in head and the max SAR averaged over 1 g in the brain induced by a lateral incident plane wave having a field strength of 0.1 V/m and induced by a mobile emitting at its mean value (50% of the max power emitted for GSM and 1% of the max power emitted for UMTS)*

The results shown in Figure 1.25 are useful to compare the typical maximum local and whole body SAR induced by up- and downlinks. However, while a mobile phone is not always used, the exposure induced by base stations is permanent. It is therefore of interest not only to compare the instantaneous value but also to perform the averaging over time.

A personal global whole body exposure (PGWBE), providing the average exposure over a time T (e.g. a month), can be defined [1.10] and can be easily extended to any organ:

$$\text{PGWBE} = \frac{1}{T}\int_0^T \text{WBSAR}(\text{posture}(t), t)_{\text{mobile}} dt + \frac{1}{T}\int_0^T \text{WBSAR}(\text{posture}(t), t)_{\text{base station}} dt \quad [1.10]$$

Equation [1.10] can be simplified if we consider:

– on the one hand, that only two postures exist (corresponding to the "voice" usage and the "data" usage) with T_1 and T_2 the time spent in emission, respectively, in "voice" and "data" usage ($T_1 + T_2 < T$);

– on the other hand, that the whole body exposure is an averaged value of the exposure associated with these two different postures.

In this case, the PGWBE over the time T can be expressed as [1.11]:

$$\text{PGWBE} = \frac{T_1}{T}\text{WBSAR}_{\text{mobile,voice}} + \frac{T_2}{T}\text{WBSAR}_{\text{mobile,data}} + \text{WBSAR}_{\text{base station}} \quad [1.11]$$

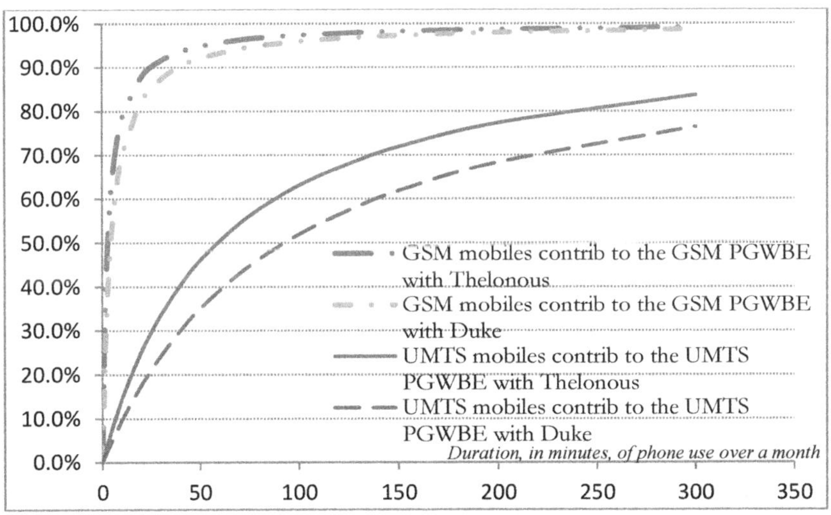

Figure 1.26. *Contribution of the mobile phone usage to the global whole body exposure versus the time (in minutes) spent on the phone per month*

The exposure induced by mobile phone usage to the PGWBE is shown in Figure 1.26. The average exposure over a time T (e.g. a month) increases with the exposure induced by the durations of use (T_1 and T_2) of the mobiles. This explains the shape of the curve showing the contribution of mobile phone usage to the global whole body exposure versus the time. Figure 1.26 also shows that the contribution of the exposure induced by UMTS phones to the PGWBE is lower than that induced by GSM phones. We can see that the exposure induced by a GSM phone is very important (more than 90% with less than 1 h), while in the case of UMTS about 200 min per month are needed to represent 80% of the global exposure.

1.2.4.4. *Global exposure and exposure index concept*

The quantities used, in European standards, to check the compliance of the exposure are the SAR and the field strength. The first, the SAR, is usually dedicated to measuring the exposure induced by sources close to the users; the second, the field strength expressed in W/m^2 (power density) or more often in V/m, is often used to quantify the exposure induced by sources far from the user, such as BSA and more generally access points. As explained in previous sections, these exposure metrics are often used with "worst-case" and consider mobile and access points separately, even if their emissions are often correlated.

Such approaches do not consider a global EMF exposure that can be defined as the averaged exposure over space and time induced by the uplink and downlink together (for a given person as well as for a population). The LEXNET project responded to existing public concerns about EMF [EUR 10] and the European Commission (EC) has specifically addressed the need for low-EMF technologies in its 7th Framework Program (FP7, ICT Call 8).

A new metric, the global index of exposure (EI), able to quantify the population exposure and taking into account the versatile use of communication system, has been defined in the FP7 LEXNET project (Low EMF Exposure Future Networks). This EI represents the average exposure of the population of the considered [LEX 12, TES 14] geographical area over the considered time frame T. The EI calculation is based on a segmentation of time period, radio access technologies, usage, etc., which depend on the objective.

The first objective of LEXNET has been to mathematically define a global EI [VAR 15] assessing the averaged exposure of the population over space and time, composed of up- and downlink sources of EMF and, as described in Figure 1.27, taking into account space, time, population, usage and technology.

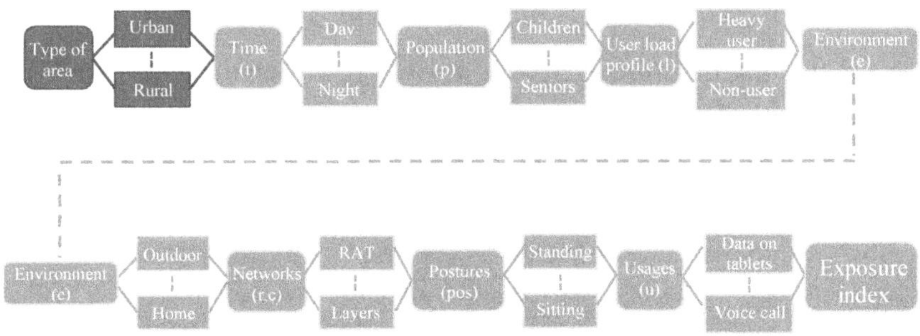

Figure 1.27. *EI definition*

The EI expressed in W/kg corresponds to the specific absorption rate averaged over the time. The EI [1.12] is a result of a transfer function of a highly complex set of data such as geographical areas, period of the day, age, networks, usages, etc., to the usual SAR metric averaged over time.

From the mathematical point of view, the EI is aggregating the uplink (ul) and down link (dl) population exposure over space and time in a single parameter using a formula [1.12] that appears complex. In fact, this is a simplistic approach but with large number of inputs and large number of sub-transfer functions:

$$\mathrm{EI} = \frac{1}{T}\sum_{\mathrm{t}}^{N_{\mathrm{T}}}\sum_{\mathrm{p}}^{N_{\mathrm{P}}}\sum_{\mathrm{e}}^{N_{\mathrm{E}}}\sum_{\mathrm{r}}^{N_{\mathrm{R}}}\sum_{\mathrm{c}}^{N_{\mathrm{C}}}\sum_{\mathrm{l}}^{N_{\mathrm{L}}}\sum_{\mathrm{pos}}^{N_{\mathrm{pos}}} f_{\mathrm{t,p,e,r,l,c,pos}}\left[\sum_{\mathrm{u}}^{N_{\mathrm{U}}}(d^{UL}\overline{\mathrm{P}}_{\mathrm{TX}}) + \mathrm{d}^{DL}\overline{\mathrm{S}}_{\mathrm{RXinc}}\right] \quad [1.12]$$

where:

– T is the period over which the EI is assessed (e.g. a day);

– N_{T} is the number of periods within the considered time frame (e.g. day, night);

– N_{P} is the number of population categories (e.g. workers, inhabitants) that have different usages;

– N_E is the number of environments (e.g. rural, urban);

– N_R is the number of radio access technologies (e.g. GSM, UMTS);

– N_C is the number of cell types (e.g. macro, microcell);

– N_L is the number of user load profiles (e.g. heavy, light);

– N_{pos} is the number of postures (e.g. standing, sitting);

– N_U is the number of usages with devices (e.g. voice, data);

– $\overline{S}_{RXinc}$ is the mean incident power density to which the human body is exposed (e.g. 2.5×10^{-5} W/m^2 with $E = 0.1$ V/m);

– $\overline{P}_{TX}$ is the mean power emitted by the users' devices during the period t, in usage mode u, connected to RATr, in environment e. In [1.12] $f_{t,p,e,r,l,c,pos}$ stands for the fraction of the population p, the user load profile l, in posture pos, connected to RAT r, for a cell type c, in the environment e during the time period t.

$\overline{S}_{RXinc}$ and $\overline{P}_{TX}$ have to be measured or estimated using planning, capacity and optimization tools [LAI 06].

In formula [1.12], d^{UL}[1.13] and d^{DL}[1.14], respectively, expressed in $\frac{Ws}{kg}/W$ (Watts per kilogram per Watt emitted) and $\frac{Ws}{kg}/\frac{W}{m^2}$ (Watts per kilogram per Watt per meter square received), stand for the normalized raw dose values for UL and DL and have to be multiplied by the time spent in the configuration:

$$d^{UL} = \frac{TD^{UL}_{t,p,l,e,r,c,u,pos} SAR^{UL}_{p,r,u,pos}}{P^{ref}_{TX}} \qquad [1.13]$$

$$d^{DL} = \frac{TD^{DL}_{t,p,e,r,c,pos} SAR^{DL}_{p,r,pos}}{S^{ref}_{RX[W]inc}} \qquad [1.14]$$

In [1.13] and [1.14], SAR stands for WBSAR as well as local averaged SAR (e.g. over an organ).

$TD^{UL}_{t,p,l,e,r,c,u,pos}$ and $TD^{DL}_{t,p,e,r,c,pos}$ represent the time duration of UL and DL exposure for an usage u, and a user profile load l, when connected to the RAT r, operating in cell type c, in the environment e, for the population category p, in the posture pos, during the time period of the day t.

$\frac{SAR^{UL}_{p,r,u,pos}}{P^{ref}_{TX}}$ and $\frac{SAR^{DL}_{p,r,pos}}{S^{ref}_{RXinc}}$ are the (whole body or organ-specific or tissue-specific as explained previously) SAR values for the usage u and the posture pos, in the frequency band of the RAT r, and the population category p, calculated, respectively, for an incident emitted power of P^{ref}_{TX} and normalized to this power and for an incident power density S^{ref}_{RXinc} and normalized to this power density. This approach has been implemented in a real configuration [VER 10] to assess the human population exposure induced in indoors and in a train for 2G (GSM 1800 MHz) and 3G (UMTS).

This concept has been also used in another paper [HUA 16], to compare the average global exposure of the population induced by macro 3G networks in different geographical areas in France and Serbia. In the latter, the input data requested by [1.12] have been collected in the different environment. For instance, the age distribution over the population (Table 1.3) and its use of information communication technologies (Table 1.4) have been analyzed. In this study, the EI linked to 3G has been estimated as 9.9×10^{-7} W/kg and 6.0×10^{-7} W/kg, respectively in French urban and suburban area, while it has been estimated, respectively, as 2.9×10^{-7} W/kg and 2.9×10^{-7} W/kg in Serbia.

Age distribution over the population	France (%)	Serbia (%)
Children	13.9	13.5
Young people	32.8	18.4
Adults	38.2	43.6
Seniors	15.1	24.5

Table 1.3. *Repartition of population in urban area of France and Serbia depending on age*

Mobile phone use		Children	Young adults	Adults	Seniors
Voice Communication	Non-user	10%	4%	5%	30%
	User	90%	96%	95%	70%
Data traffic	Non-user	45%	33%	59%	90%
	User	55%	67%	41%	10%

Table 1.4. *Proportions of users and non-users of mobile phones per population category*

$\overline{S}_{RXinc}$ and $\overline{P}_{TX}$, used in [1.12], are often estimated using planning, capacity and optimization tools. The usual deterministic propagation prediction methods used to design the network and estimate the capacity generally fail to accommodate the human body. They usually consider a constant body loss and an isotropic gain for the user device. In fact, the gain of the couple composed of the user's body and the user's device is not isotropic as shown in section 2.4.3.1. Assuming a constant noise power at the receiver location, keeping the SNR [THO 91] close to the target will require that the power emitted by the phone varies inversely to the variations of the gain, in order to have the received power at the base stational most constant. As a consequence, the position of the phone relatively to the body will influence, on the one hand, the normalized quantity $\frac{SAR^{UL}_{p,r,u,pos}}{P^{ref}_{TX}}$ and, on the other hand, power emitted $\overline{P}_{TX}$ (see section 2.4.3.1).

1.3. European standards and regulation framework

In Europe and in the RF exposure domain, the regulation framework is composed of three parts. The first recommends the human health protection limits that have to be used; the second establishes the methods and protocols that can be (or will be) used to check the compliance of systems put on the market or put into service. The last component, at the European or at the National level, is the directive or the law providing the legal requirements.

On the subject of limits, the World Health Organization[1] (WHO) and the Committee on Protection against Non-Ionizing Radiation Protection[2] (ICNIRP) have defined levels of protection of people against over-exposure induced by EMFs. In Europe, the European Scientific Toxico-Ecological Committee (CSTEE)[3] of Europe has confirmed the ICNIRP guidelines.

The EC gives the legal framework. On July 12, 1999, the EC issued a recommendation (1999/519/EC)[4] based on ICNIRP and CSTEE opinions.

---

1 www.who.int.
2 www.icnirp.org.
3 http://ec.europa.eu/health/scientific_committees/environmental_risks/sctee/index_en.htm.
4 http://ec.europa.eu/health/electromagnetic_fields/docs/emf_rec519_en.pdf.

This latter has been transposed in national regulation as in France in 2002 with a decree dated May 3, 2002 (decree no. 2002-775)[5].

In Europe, as explained in the introduction of this section, equipment that intentionally emits or receives radiowaves for the purpose of radio communication have to comply with the R&TTE European directive [DIR 14]. In 2016, a new directive 2014/53/EU [DIR 99] (known as RED) is replacing this R&TTE directive but the main objectives are similar. They lead to put on the market and put into service equipment and devices that satisfy essential requirements that in the RF exposure domain are provided by the European council recommendation.

The European system for technical standardization is composed of CENELEC (www.cenelec.eu), ETSI (www.etsi.org) and CEN (www.cen.eu) that are, respectively, responsible for European standardization in the area of electrical engineering, telecommunications and other technical areas. The documents ratified by one of these three European Standards are the European Standards (EN). In the field of telecommunications, most technical standards are issued under the auspices of ETSI. Regarding health issues in the essential requirements relating to directive RTTE, the EC has given the mandate (M035). One of the CENELEC technical committees, the CENELEC TC 106[6], is dealing with various aspects of the exposure of people to EMFs from 0 Hz to 300 GHz.

To help entities legally responsible for putting equipment onto the market or into service, the Commission has given a mandate to CENELEC (M035) to develop a set of standards, the "harmonized standards", that can be used to check product compliance with the requirements. The products that are compliant with the requirement of these standards are deemed to comply with the essential requirements requested by the RED.

The standards, including the harmonized standards, produced by CENELEC are of three different types: product, generic and basic. The product standards provide the presumption of conformity of product put on

5 http://www.legifrance.gouv.fr/affichTexte.do?cidTexte=JORFTEXT000000226401

6 http://www.cenelec.eu/dyn/www/f?p=104:7:1747965399249801:FSP_ORG_ID,FSP_LANG_ID:1258483,25

the market or into service, they define the requirements and test methods that have to be used for a coherent range of products.

The basic standards provide standardized test methods, the technical basic requirements and guidance (including background). The basic standards do not by themselves provide a presumption of conformity but are referenced in the product standards.

The generic standards are dedicated to the compliance tests of products for which product standards have not been developed. In this case, the generic standards define the requirements, test methods and protocols that have to be used to check the compliance. Conversely to the product standard, the generic standards are based on types of environment rather than product categories.

For mobile and base stations, the TC 106x working group has finalized and presented seven standards. The first set of standards, published in the official journal of the EC in 2001, were composed of basic and product standards (respectively, EN50360 and EN50361). The second set of basic and product standards dedicated to put on the market of base stations is composed of EN50383 and EN50384 and has been published in in the official journal of the EC in 2002. The third set is composed of the product and basics standards dedicated to put into service the base stations (EN50400 and EN50401). The last one is only a technical standard dedicated to the *in situ* measurement of EMF (EN50492).

Worldwide, the IEC (www.iec.ch) is also preparing and publishing International Standards for all electrical, electronic and related technologies collectively. To avoid a duplication of efforts, and to reduce time when preparing standard and facilitate coherence between the European and the international standards in the electrical sector, CENELEC and IEC formalized in 1996 a framework of cooperation, known as the Dresden Agreement[7]. In coherence with this agreement, the maintenance and follow up of the European basic standard have been transferred to IEC. Today, EN62209-1 and EN62209-2 have replaced EN50360, and IEC is working toward a standard covering the basic requirement of EN50383, EN50400 and EN50492.

7 ftp://ftp.cencenelec.eu/CENELEC/Guides/CLC/13_CENELECGuide13.pdf

1.4. Conclusion

In this chapter, we have analyzed the metric and limits relative to human exposure. The human RF exposure, the SAR, the protection limits and the basic restrictions have been defined. The relationship between the basic restrictions and the reference levels has been explained. This chapter has also described the exposure assessment for compliance test and the European standardization framework dedicated to the compliance analysis. The real power emitted by the systems has been described and the new concept of an exposure index has been introduced.

As described in this chapter, the SAR measurement is not only complex but also invasive. Because of this, numerical dosimetry is complementing the experimental approach to have the SAR distribution in tissues and organs. The next chapter will introduce numerical dosimetry, analyze the numerical method to assess the exposure and will provide examples of applications.

2

Computational Electromagnetics Applied to Human Exposure Assessment

"It takes imagination to represent reality".

Giuseppe PONTIGGIA

2.1. Introduction

Taking advantage of recent progresses in high-performance calculation (HPC) based on, for example, parallel architectures or/and graphic processors units (GPU), large efforts are being made today to develop numerical methods that can be used to assess the radio frequency (RF) exposure [IEE 15a, IEE 15b]. The computational techniques have taken advantage of these progresses; commercial codes based on various approaches such as the finite element method (FEM) or finite difference in time domain (FDTD) are available nowadays and their uses are not only dedicated to specialist researchers or engineers. In the RF domain, due to the increasing use of wireless communication systems, questions about risk perception and possible health impacts linked to RF have led, because of the progress in HPC, to using the FDTD to design systems and assess human exposure. This chapter discusses exposure modeling and presents case studies that show the ability of this method to assess the human exposure induced by RF sources. It presents case studies in the near field and at larger distances using equivalent principles and spherical mode expansion of RF sources.

2.2. Finite difference in time domain to solve the Maxwell equations

2.2.1. *Introduction*

There is a large literature dealing with the FDTD method [TAL 95, KUN 93]. The objective of this section is therefore not to duplicate what exists elsewhere. The aim is to point out and discuss the key points of FDTD that is nowadays the most popular method in bio-electromagnetism. The complexity of wireless communication systems and the strong heterogeneity of human tissues lead to very large problems from a computational point of view. As an example, human exposure assessment using numerical methods and a human phantom model [ACK 95] having a millimeter resolution can involve a few million unknowns. The FDTD, by construction, does not require any matrix inversion and can handle such large problems. This advantage and the simplicity of the method has led to use intensively the FDTD in bio-electromagnetics. Before pointing out some questions specific to this domain, we will first summarize the main principle of the methods.

The well-known Maxwell [JAM 65, JAM 04] equations govern the relationship between the electric and magnetic components of the electromagnetic field (EMF). In case of non-dispersive, isotropic, heterogeneous and lossy media, these relationships in time domain between the electric field $\vec{E}\left(\overrightarrow{M(x,y,z)},t\right)$ and the magnetic field $\vec{H}\left(\overrightarrow{M(x,y,z)},t\right)$ are given by the equations [2.1] and [2.2].

$$\overrightarrow{\mathrm{rot}\left(E(x,y,z,t)\right)} = -\mu(x,y,z)\frac{\partial \overrightarrow{H(x,y,z,t)}}{\partial t} \qquad [2.1]$$

$$\overrightarrow{\mathrm{rot}\left(H(x,y,z,t)\right)} = +\varepsilon(x,y,z)\frac{\partial \overrightarrow{E(x,y,z,t)}}{\partial t} + \overrightarrow{J(x,y,z,t)} \qquad [2.2]$$

In these equations, M represents the point of coordinates (x, y, z), t the time, ε the permittivity and μ the permeability of the media at coordinates (x, y, z). These equations can have analytical solutions such as plane waves or spherical waves in specific configurations but most of the time they do not have analytical solution in case of complex media. Because of that, the solutions are often obtained using numerical calculation.

The FDTD is based on a sampling of the electric and magnetic fields vectors $\vec{E}(x, y, z, t)$ & $\vec{H}(x, y, z, t)$ over a time and space grid [YEE 66] often orthogonal but not always [TAF 95, GIL 00]. With this method, the vectors $\vec{E}$ and $\vec{H}$ are represented through six matrices $\{E_x, E_y, E_z, H_x, H_y, H_z\}$ of their component sampled at different points x_i, y_i, z_i and t_i. The vector components may be co-located or not [GIL 00]. Among the possible patterns of discretization, some are implicit and require matrix inversion that does not allow for handling very large problems. Some patterns are explicit and can be used to solve the Maxwell equation through an iterative process that does not need any matrix inversion but requires complying with some constraints in order to be stable. The pattern of sampling also influences the accuracy of the derivative approximation of equation [2.3]. The non-centered differences provide a first-order accuracy; the centered finite differences have a big advantage in the field of waves since, as shown by [2.3] and [2.4], they provide a second-order accuracy of the derivative estimation.

$$f(x_0 \pm h/2) = f(x_0) \pm \frac{\partial f}{\partial x}(x_0)\left[\frac{h}{2}\right] + \frac{\partial^2 f}{\partial x^2}(x_0)\left[\frac{h^2}{4}\right] + \mathcal{O}(h^2) \qquad [2.3]$$

$$\overrightarrow{\mathrm{rot}(H(x, y, z, t)} = +\varepsilon(x, y, z)\frac{\partial \overrightarrow{E(x,y,z,t)}}{\partial t} + \overrightarrow{J(x, y, z, t)} \qquad [2.4]$$

A higher order scheme can be used [DEV 92] but the computational effort is much more important. Indeed, the higher order scheme involves the E and H components not only of the surrounding cells but also those of more distant cells.

In exposure assessment, the centered differences are often used in areas of main interest to keep the accuracy at a high level while non-centered differences are used for other areas allowing us, in this way, to significantly reduce the memory requirement [WIA 98]. The trade-off is in this case between the accuracy and the memory, even if today the memory constraints are less important than they were in the past.

The most popular FDTD scheme is the YEE scheme [YEE 66] with the sampling as shown in Figure 2.1. As explained previously, the components of E and H vectors can be sampled at different locations and times; one requirement for keeping the second-order accuracy is to assess the equality of discretized derivative involved in [2.1] and [2.2] at the same space and time location. This approach implies an intertwining sampling known as "leap frog" (see Figure 2.2).

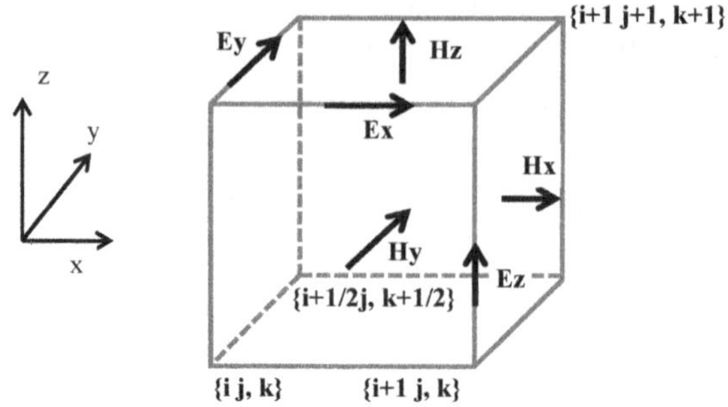

Figure 2.1. *Yee cell with the location of the E and H components*

Consider the 1D version. With Δx as the grid step and Δt as the time step, the leap frog approach leads to the sample of E performed at $\left(i+\frac{1}{2}\right)\Delta x$ and $(k)\,\Delta t$, while the sample of H is performed $(i)\,\Delta x$ and $\left(k+\frac{1}{2}\right)\Delta t$ allowing us to have a centered approach and a collocation of the derivatives:

$$\frac{E\left(x+\frac{\Delta x}{2},t\right)-E\left(x-\frac{\Delta x}{2},t\right)}{\Delta x}=-\mu\frac{H\left(x,t+\frac{\Delta t}{2}\right)-H\left(x,t-\frac{\Delta t}{2}\right)}{\Delta t} \quad [2.5]$$

$$\frac{H\left(x,t-\frac{\Delta t}{2}\right)-H\left(x-\Delta x,t-\frac{\Delta t}{2}\right)}{\Delta x}=\varepsilon\frac{E\left(x-\frac{\Delta x}{2},t\right)-E\left(x-\frac{\Delta x}{2},t-\Delta t\right)}{\Delta t} \quad [2.6]$$

In 3D and using a uniform orthogonal grid, the components of E and H vectors are located, as shown in Figure 2.1, on the edge and on the face of a cube known as a "Yee cell" since it was proposed by Yee in 1966 [YEE 66]. As pointed out previously, the components of E and H vectors are also sampled at a time having a half time step difference.

$$Ex^{n}_{i,j,k}=E_x\left(\left(i-\frac{1}{2}\right)dx,jdy,kdz,ndt\right) \quad [2.7]$$

$$Ey^{n}_{i,j,k}=E_y\left(idx,\left(j-\frac{1}{2}\right)dy,kdz,ndt\right)$$

$$Ez^{n}_{i,j,k}=E_x\left(idx,jdy,\left(k-\frac{1}{2}\right)dz,ndt\right);$$

$$Hx_{i,j,k}^{n} = H_x\left(idx, \left(j - \frac{1}{2}\right)dy, \left(k - \frac{1}{2}\right)dz, \left(n + \frac{1}{2}\right)dt\right)$$

$$Hy_{i,j,k}^{n} = H_x\left(\left(i - \frac{1}{2}\right)dx, jdy, \left(k - \frac{1}{2}\right)dz, \left(n + \frac{1}{2}\right)dt\right)$$

$$Hz_{i,j,k}^{n} = H_z\left(\left(i - \frac{1}{2}\right)dx, \left(j - \frac{1}{2}\right)dy, kdz, \left(n + \frac{1}{2}\right)dt\right)$$

Using the notation given in [2.7], the relation provided in [2.5] and [2.6] can be rewritten as in [2.8]. With β and γ coefficients derived from [2.5] and [2.6],

$$E_i^{n+1} = E_i^n + \beta[H_{i+1}^n - H_i^n] \qquad [2.8]$$

$$H_i^{n+1} = H_i^n + \gamma\left[E_i^{n+1} - E_i^{n+1}\right]$$

REMARK.– As discussed previously, non-centered differences can also be used, even if in this case the accuracy is lower. In this case, the grid size $\{dx_i, dy_j, dz_k\}$ depends on the location and cannot be considered as constant as in [2.7]. Using these notations, equations [2.6] and [2.7] and the leap frog approach lead to the explicit formulation that is described graphically in Figure 2.2.

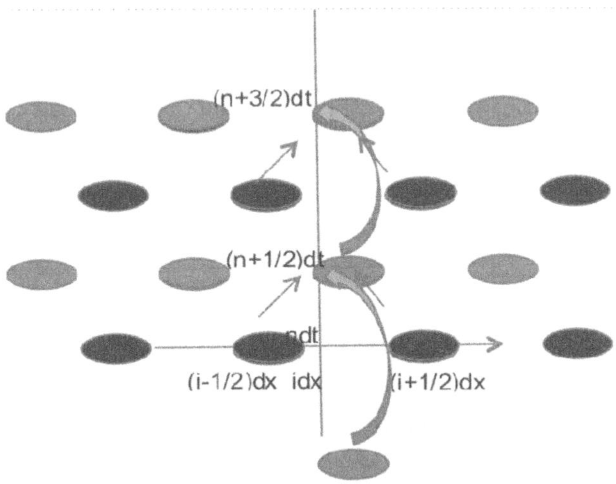

Figure 2.2. *Leap frog scheme of the FDTD calculation. For a color version of the figure, see www.iste.co.uk/wiart/radiofrequency.zip*

Solving the Maxwell equations using the present approach is efficient but is conditionally stable. The following section will discuss the stability condition that time and spatial steps have to comply with in order to allow a stable solver. The immediate question following the stability is the accuracy. While a non-stable scheme is of course inaccurate, a stable solver can also be inaccurate. Related to the accuracy is the question of the influence of the finite grid on the wave propagation and signal dispersion.

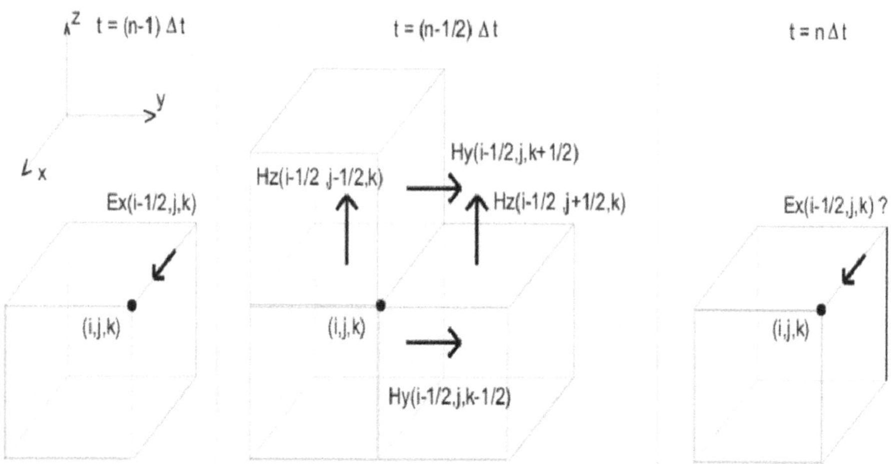

Figure 2.3. *FDTD scheme*

In 3D, for homogeneous and lossless media the FDTD expressions involve E and H components. For instance, derived from previous equations and notations, E_x is given by [2.9]:

$$E_{x_{i,j,k}}^{\,n+1} = E_{x_{i,j,k}}^{\,n} + \frac{dt}{\varepsilon}\left[\frac{\left(H_{z_{i,j+1,k}}^{\,n} - H_{z_{i,j,k}}^{\,n}\right)}{dy} - \frac{\left(H_{y_{i,j,k+1}}^{\,n} - H_{y_{i,j,k}}^{\,n}\right)}{dz}\right] \qquad [2.9]$$

In case of lossy dielectric media, equation [2.2] translated in the "FDTD" algorithm involves the E field at time ndt and $(n+1)dt$ as shown in equation [2.9] but also the current J at $\left(n+\frac{1}{2}\right)dt$ (as H). Equation [2.10] gives the relation between the current J, the conductivity σ and the electric field E.

$$\overrightarrow{J(x,y,z,t)} = \sigma(x,y,z)\overrightarrow{E(x,y,z,t)} \qquad [2.10]$$

We can see that [2.10] needs to have the E field at time sample $(n + \frac{1}{2})dt$ that only exists for the H field. To overcome this problem, the E field at time $(n + \frac{1}{2})dt$ has to be derived from known values at ndt and $(n + 1)dt$ [2.11]

$$E^{n+\frac{1}{2}} = (E^{n+1} + E^{n})/2 . \qquad [2.11]$$

The combination of [2.2], [2.9], [2.10] and [2.11] provides new equations whilst taking into account the current ones. Equation [2.12] gives the new updating of the *x* component of the electric field.

$$E_{x\,i,j,k}^{\,n+1} = \left[\frac{1-\sigma dt/_{2\varepsilon}}{1+\sigma dt/_{2\varepsilon}}\right] + \frac{dt/_{\varepsilon}}{1+\sigma dt/_{2\varepsilon}}\left[\frac{\left(H_{z\,i,j+1,k}^{\,n}-H_{z\,i,j,k}^{\,n}\right)}{dy} - \frac{\left(H_{y\,i,j,k+1}^{\,n}-H_{y\,i,j,k}^{\,n}\right)}{dz}\right] \qquad [2.12]$$

2.2.2. *Stability, dispersion and accuracy*

2.2.2.1. *Stability*

Large efforts have been carried to get a stable pattern. For the FDTD, the main contributions are those of Courant, Friedrichs and Lewy (CFL) [COU 28] who have proposed a stability through a relationship [2.13] between the time and spatial steps dt , dx, dy, dz.

$$dt \le \frac{1}{v\sqrt{\frac{1}{dx^2}+\frac{1}{dy^2}+\frac{1}{dz^2}}} \qquad [2.13]$$

where v is the light velocity in the media. In the case of a non-uniform grid, $\{dx_i, dy_j, dz_k\}$ are not constant over the grid and the stability is therefore achieved with $dt \le \min_{\{i,j,k\}}\left[\frac{1}{v\sqrt{\frac{1}{(dx_i)^2}+\frac{1}{(dy_j)^2}+\frac{1}{(dz_k)^2}}}\right]$.

2.2.2.2. *Dispersion and numerical velocity*

Consider an electromagnetic wave propagating in a homogeneous and infinite medium. The electric field has to comply with the well-known equation [2.14]

$$\nabla^2\vec{E} = \frac{1}{v^2}\frac{\partial^2\vec{E}}{\partial t^2} \qquad [2.14]$$

where ∇ is the well-known "Nabla" operator, t the time and ν the light velocity in the media. Let us consider a plane wave having a pulsation ω and let us note $\vec{k} = (k_x, k_y, k_z)$ the propagation vector. The electric field is then defined as [2.15]

$$\vec{E}(t,x,y,z) = \overrightarrow{E_0} e^{j\omega t} e^{-j(k_x x + k_y y + k_z z)} \qquad [2.15]$$

To be able to propagate in the media, the E field has to comply with the propagation equation [2.14] that imposes that $\{\vec{k}, \omega, \nu\}$ comply with the dispersion equation given by:

$$\frac{\omega^2}{\nu^2} = k_x^2 + k_y^2 + k_z^2 \qquad [2.16]$$

To perform simulations, the equation is discretized over a grid. Consider a uniform grid $\{\Delta x, \Delta y, \Delta z, \Delta t\}$, then the plane wave equation in the grid is given by:

$$\vec{E}(n,i,j,k) = \overrightarrow{E_0} e^{j\omega n\Delta t} e^{-jk_x\, i\Delta x - jk_y j\Delta y - jk_z k\Delta z)} \qquad [2.17]$$

$$\frac{\sin^2\left[\omega\frac{(\Delta t)^2}{2}\right]}{c^2(\Delta t)^2} = \frac{\sin^2\left[k_x\frac{(\Delta x)^2}{2}\right]}{(\Delta x)^2} + \frac{\sin^2\left[k_y\frac{(\Delta y)^2}{2}\right]}{(\Delta y)^2} + \frac{\sin^2\left[k_z\frac{(\Delta z)^2}{2}\right]}{(\Delta z)^2} \qquad [2.18]$$

The phase and group velocities of a wave are defined, respectively, as the rate at which the phase and the shape of the amplitudes propagate in space. Because of the discretization of the space, these velocities depend on the grid step. In 2D and using the grid step $\Delta x = \Delta y = \Delta$, the phase velocity can be derived, using Newton's method, for instance, from [2.18]. Figure 2.4 shows the results for various angles and grid size normalized to wavelength (i.e. $\frac{\Delta}{\lambda}$) in the media.

As shown in Figure 2.4, a FDTD grid size close to $\lambda/_{10}$ provides quite a good result and this resolution is often used in FDTD simulation. In case of heterogeneous tissues the "$\lambda/_{10}$" target has to be achieved in all the tissues. For instance, at the frequency of 900 MHz the relative permittivity of brain white matter, muscle and cerebro-spinal-fluid (often known as CSF) are[1] respectively 38, 55 and 68. In these tissues the wavelengths are respectively 4.8 cm, 4 cm and 3.6 cm. The permittivity of the CSF is the highest then the

1 http://niremf.ifac.cnr.it/tissprop/.

target grid size is 3 mm, at 5 GHz the CSF relative permittivity is 62 so the target grid size is 0.7 mm. If the same object is modeled, then the memory request at 5 GHz will be more than 64 times higher than the memory requested at 900 MHz.

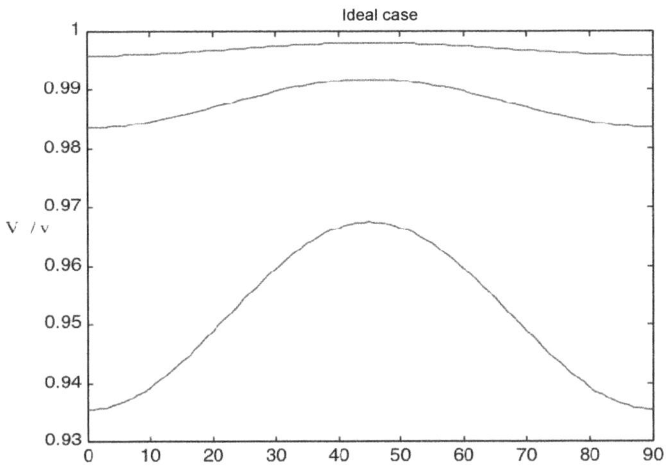

Figure 2.4. $\frac{v_\varphi}{v}$ *versus angle for grid size normalized to the wavelength. λ/20 (upper), λ /10 (middle) , λ /5 (lower)*

2.2.3. *Boundary conditions*

Because of the memory, the computational domain is limited and boundary conditions are necessary to perform a truncation without creating artifacts into the computation of the E and H fields. These boundary conditions are composed of rules to set the values of E and H at the edge of the grid. For instance, a simple Dirichlet boundary condition sets the E field solution to zero at the edge of the grid (in this case, as a perfect metal acts, the edge of the grid is reflecting the waves that hit itself). Most of the time, the objective is not to assess the exposure of a person located in a metallic box but to avoid any spurious reflection at the borders. The objective of absorbing boundary conditions (ABCs) is (as shown in Figure 2.5) to keep outgoing E and H fields from being reflected back into the domain of simulation.

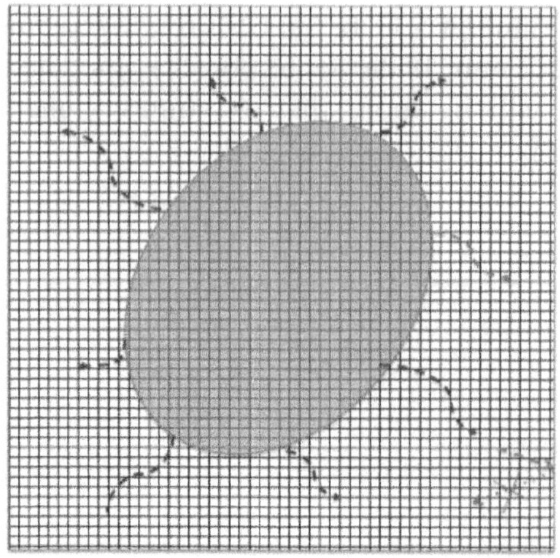

Figure 2.5. *Schema of a typical absorbing condition aiming to avoid refection at the boundary of the computational domain*

As described in Figure 2.6, the calculation of the E field at the border requires [2.9] to have not only the H field inside the computational domain but also outside. The challenge is therefore to extrapolate from the field calculated in the computational field the value outside of this domain.

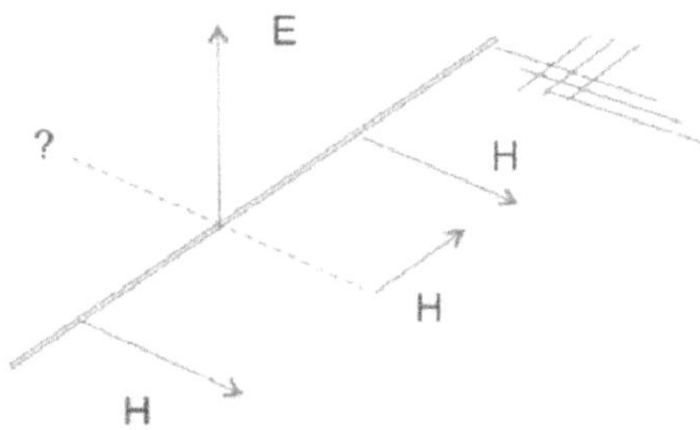

Figure 2.6. *Missing values at the limits of the computational domain*

As a first approach, the first-order "MUR" conditions (introduced by Mur [MUR 81]) are easy to describe in 1D: they consider that the wave at the boundary follows equation [2.19].

$$\left[\frac{\partial^2}{\partial x^2} - \frac{\partial^2}{c^2\,\partial t^2}\right]\left(E_{Z_{x=0}}\right) = 0 = \left(\frac{\partial}{\partial x} - \frac{\partial}{c\,\partial t}\right)\left(\frac{\partial}{\partial x} + \frac{\partial}{c\,\partial t}\right)\left(E_{Z_{x=0}}\right) \qquad [2.19]$$

that are satisfied if

$$\left(\frac{\partial}{\partial x}-\frac{\partial}{c\,\partial t}\right)\left(E_{Z_{x=0}}\right)=0 \qquad [2.20]$$

At the boundary, equations [2.5] and [2.6] can be replaced by equation [2.21] that expresses in the grid equation [2.20]:

$$E_z^{n+1}(i,j,k)=E_z^{n+1}(i+1,j,k)+\frac{c\Delta t-\Delta x}{c\Delta t+\Delta x}\left[E_z^{n+1}(i+1,j,k)-E_z^{n}(i+1,j,k)\right] \qquad [2.21]$$

Another approach is to absorb the out-coming wave. The perfect matching layers [BER 94], known as PMLs, created ABCs toward this objective. Today, PMLs are the most accurate and used ABC methods.

Consider a transverse electric (TE) wave $\{(E_x, E_y, 0); (0,0,H_z)\}$ propagating from free space $(\varepsilon_0\mu_0)$ to the lossy medium $\{(\varepsilon_0,\sigma)(\mu_0,\sigma^*)\}$.

$$\varepsilon_0\frac{\partial E_x}{\partial t}+\sigma E_x=\frac{\partial H_z}{\partial y} \qquad [2.22]$$

$$\varepsilon_0\frac{\partial E_y}{\partial t}+\sigma E_y=-\frac{\partial H_z}{\partial x} \qquad [2.23]$$

$$\mu_0\frac{\partial H_z}{\partial t}+\sigma^* H_z=\frac{\partial E_x}{\partial y}-\frac{\partial E_y}{\partial x} \qquad [2.24]$$

In this case, the complex medium impedance of this media is, respectively, given by:

$$\mu=\sqrt{\frac{\mu_0}{\varepsilon_0}} \quad \text{and} \quad \mu^*=\sqrt{\frac{\mu_0-\frac{j\sigma^*}{\omega}}{\varepsilon_0-\frac{j\sigma}{\omega}}}=\sqrt{\frac{\mu_0}{\varepsilon_0}}\left[\sqrt{\frac{1-\frac{j\sigma^*}{\mu_0\omega}}{1-\frac{j\sigma}{\varepsilon_0\omega}}}\right] \qquad [2.25]$$

When the dielectric properties of the media follow [2.26], then the media have the same impedance. They are matched and there is no reflection for the TE wave at the boundary.

$$\frac{\sigma^*}{\mu_0}=\frac{\sigma}{\varepsilon_0} \qquad [2.26]$$

This property has been used by Berenger, who introduced the PML in 1994 [BER 94]. The latter are composed of artificial material and are able to absorb the out-coming wave, having an arbitrary angle and therefore avoiding reflections at the boundaries. Than original approach is often called the "split PML", because the waves are artificially split into two artificial non-Maxwellian field components [MAX 95]. The approach has been revisited with uniaxial PMLs (UPMLs) [SAC 95] that allow us, with a combination of artificial anisotropic absorbing materials, to express the PML region as an ordinary region. Both UPMLs and "split" PMLs can be also viewed as the results of a complex coordinate stretching [CHE 94]. Using such a complex coordinate approach, the fields exponentially decay along the complex spatial coordinate.

2.2.4. *FDTD approach to thin wires and layers*

2.2.4.1. *Introduction*

Modeling with a description of the volume and a thin wire may require a very large memory with FDTD. For instance, with a grid mesh 1 mm in size (that represents, in free space, 3% of the wavelength at 900 MHz) taking into account a wire of 0.1 mm, will increase the memory requirement by 1,000 and the computation time by 10,000. In the electromagnetic compatibility, the coupling to wire structure is a key question; because of this larger efforts [HOL 81, BER 00, BRE 89, EDE 03, GUI 12] have been conducted to efficiently model thin wire. The same limit exists with thin layers. The main idea is modify the E and H field components calculated in the FDTD cells to take into account the presence of a thin wire or thin layer (i.e. typically smaller than a tenth of the cell size) that exists but is not modeled in the FDTD grid.

2.2.4.2. *Thin wires*

The first approach, based on the E field property in perfect electrical conductors (PECs), consists of putting the E field components to zero, as shown in Figure 2.7, located in the wire. Such an approach is also used to model metal structures.

The second approach is of great interest because of the parsimony but does not take into account the E field properties in the vicinity of such a thin wire. An advanced method [TAF 95] consists of putting constraints not only on the E field component located in the thin wire but also on the radial and the ortho-radial components of the electric and magnetic fields in the vicinity of the wire. Assuming that the wire is aligned with the x axis, then the E_y

and H_x components are inversely proportional to the distance to the wire (*y* axis in Figure 2.8).

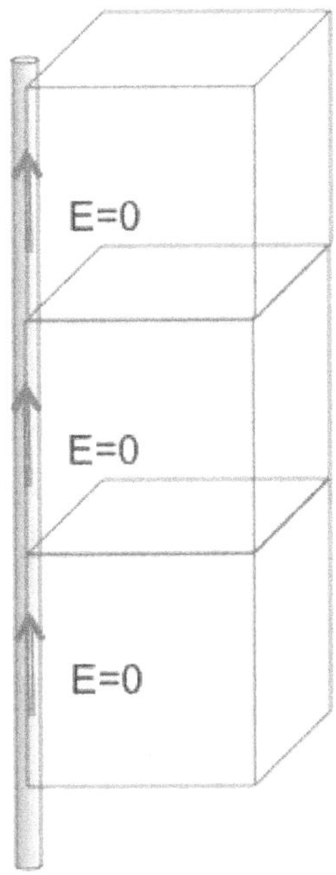

Figure 2.7. *PEC thin wire approach forcing the E field to zero*

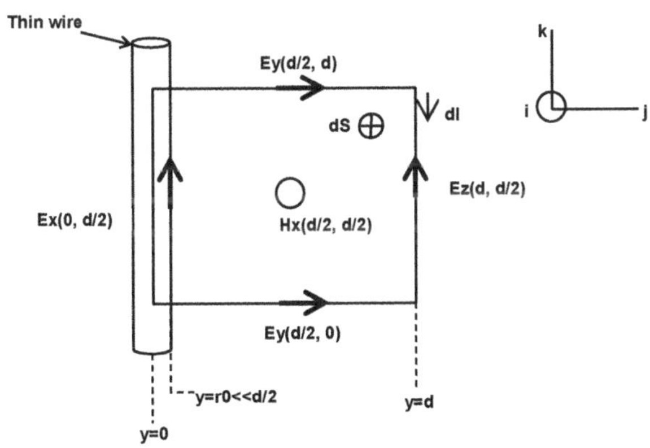

Figure 2.8. *Thin wire approach used by Taflove [TAF 95]*

With the notations of Figure 2.8, the properties of the EMF are given by equations [2.27]–[2.30].

$$H_x(y,z) = H_x\left(\tfrac{d}{2},\tfrac{d}{2}\right)\left[1 - c_1\left(z - \tfrac{d}{2}\right)\right]\frac{\frac{d}{2}}{y} \qquad [2.27]$$

$$E_y(0 \text{ or } d, y) = E_y\left(0 \text{ or } d, \tfrac{d}{2}\right)\frac{\frac{d}{2}}{y} \qquad [2.28]$$

$$E_z(0,z) = 0 \qquad [2.29]$$

$$E_z(d,z) = E_z\left(d,\tfrac{d}{2}\right)\ \left[1 - c_2\left(z - \tfrac{d}{2}\right)\right] \qquad [2.30]$$

In these equations, c_1 and c_2 are constants that are not required to be known for this purpose. Using the Maxwell–Faraday law ($\oint_\tau \vec{E}(\vec{r},t)d\vec{l} = -\mu\frac{\partial}{\partial t}\iint_S \vec{H}(\vec{r},t)d\vec{l}$), the surface described in Figure 2.8 and equations [2.27]–[2.30], the H_x, H_y, H_z components can be expressed in the FDTD scheme as H_x in [2.31].

$$\begin{aligned} H_x^{n+\frac{1}{2}}(d/2,d/2) = H_x^{n-\frac{1}{2}}(d/2,d/2) &- \frac{\Delta t}{\mu_0}\cdot\frac{1}{\frac{d}{2}\ln\frac{d}{r_0}}\left[E_z^n(d,d/2) - 0\right] \\ &+ \frac{\Delta t}{\mu_0}\cdot\frac{1}{d}\left[E_y^n(d/2,d) - E_y^n(d/2,0)\right] \end{aligned} \qquad [2.31]$$

where d is the FDTD cell size and r_0 the radius of the thin wire. The main limit of this approach is linked to the wire location that is aligned with the grid. This approach has been improved [HOL 81] using a pseudo-hybrid approach of the FDTD and the line equation taking into account, on the one hand (as in the previous method), the inverse dependency of the radial and ortho-radial components E and H fields [2.32] to the distance to the wire (see Figure 2.9) and, on the other hand, the linear charge Q and the current I of the wire [2.33]:

$$H_\theta(r) = \frac{I}{2\pi r} \text{ and } E_r(r) = \frac{Q}{2\pi r\varepsilon_0} \qquad [2.32]$$

$$\frac{\partial Q(s,t)}{\partial t} + \frac{\partial I(s,t)}{\partial s} = 0 \qquad [2.33]$$

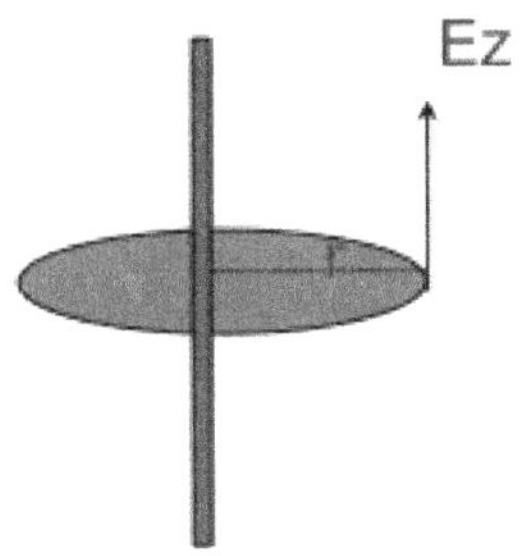

Figure 2.9. *Holland approach of the thin wire*

One of the Maxwell equations in a cylindrical coordinate is given by:

$$\frac{\partial E_r}{\partial z} - \frac{\partial E_z}{\partial r} = -\mu\left[\frac{\partial H_\theta}{\partial t}\right] \qquad [2.34]$$

The integration of [2.34] along a radius $[r_0, r]$ gives [2.35]:

$$\int_{r_0}^{r} \frac{\partial E_r}{\partial z} dr - \int_{r_0}^{r} \frac{\partial E_z}{\partial r} dr = -\mu_0 \frac{\partial}{\partial t} \int_{r_0}^{r} H_\theta dr \qquad [2.35]$$

The combination of [2.32] and [2.35] provides [2.36] and [2.37] that is a new time and space relationship between E, Q and I:

$$\int_{r_0}^{r} \frac{\partial E_z}{\partial r} dr = \frac{1}{2\pi\varepsilon_0} \frac{\partial Q}{\partial z} \int_{r_0}^{r} \frac{1}{r} dr + \frac{\mu_0}{2\pi} \frac{\partial I}{\partial t} \int_{r_0}^{r} \frac{1}{r} dr \qquad [2.36]$$

$$<E_z(r)> = < \frac{1}{2\pi\varepsilon_0} \ln\left(\frac{r}{r_0}\right) > \left[\frac{\partial Q}{\partial z} + \varepsilon_0\mu_0 \frac{\partial I}{\partial t}\right] \qquad [2.37]$$

A first approach [HOL 81] has been to average [2.37] on a constant area (e.g. the Yee cell or a cylinder) that leads to get

$$\frac{\partial I(s,t)}{\partial t} + c^2 \frac{\partial Q(s,t)}{\partial s} = \frac{< E(s,t) >}{L} \qquad [2.38]$$

where L is the linear inductance. If we consider the averaging over a disk having a radius $R = \sqrt{\Delta_x^2 + \Delta_y^2}$, then L is given by [2.39]:

$$L = \frac{1}{R} \iint \frac{1}{2\pi\varepsilon_0} \ln\left(\frac{r}{r_0}\right) dr \sim \frac{1}{2\pi\varepsilon_0} \ln\left(\frac{R}{r_0}\right) \qquad [2.39]$$

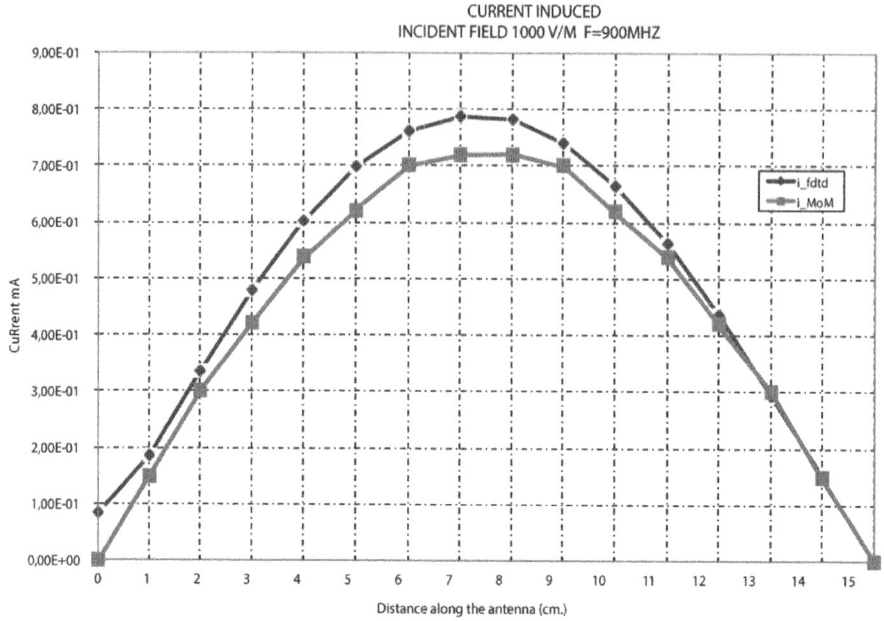

Figure 2.10. *Comparison of current in wire induced by an incident wave (900 MHz, 1,000 v/m) assessed with on the one hand the FDTD and the wire modeled using the "Holland" approach, on the other hand the moment method (MoM)*

As shown in Figure 2.10, large efforts have been carried out in the 1990s on thin wire including multi-wire [BER 00] and oblique formalism [EDE 03, FDT 12] but this formalism is nowadays more relevant to electromagnetic compatibility than to exposure assessment. Indeed, the grid size used in SAR calculation is often close to the millimeter and the thin wire modeling is less used since patch antennas are nowadays often used in handheld mobile phone.

2.2.4.3. *Thin layer*

The "thin layer" modeling objective is similar to the "thin wire" one. The idea is to modify the E and H field component calculated in the FDTD cells to take into account the presence of a thin layer that exists but is not modeled in the FDTD grid.

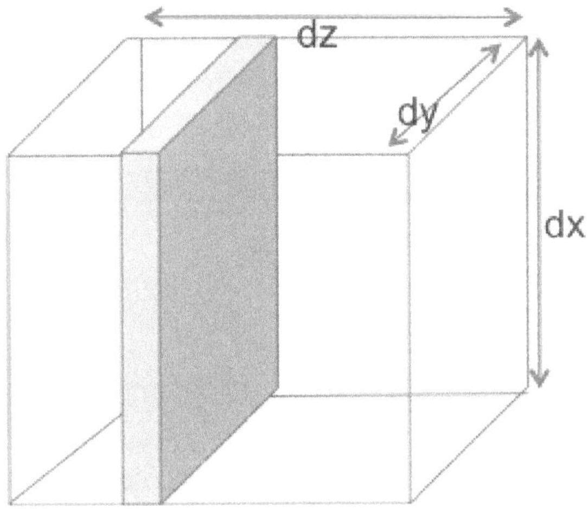

Figure 2.11. *Example of a thin layer in the FDTD Yee cell*

In the case of a PEC thin layer, the simplest approach is to force the E field tangential component to zero. This method is similar to thin wire modeling.

In the case of a non-PEC layer, another approach is requested. Let us consider a layer as shown in Figure 2.11 with Δ as thickness, $\{\varepsilon, \sigma, \mu\}$ the dielectric properties in the cell and $\{\varepsilon', \sigma', \mu\}$ in the layer. In the Yee cell the relationship between E and H are governed by Maxwell equations [2.1] and [2.2]. Let us consider a surface S and the contour δ of this surface. The integration of the [2.1] and [2.2] over the surface S gives

$$\iint_S \overrightarrow{\mathrm{rot}(\vec{E})} d\vec{s} = \oint_\delta \vec{E} d\vec{l} = -\mu \frac{\partial}{\partial t} \iint_S \vec{H} d\vec{s} \qquad [2.40]$$

$$\iint_S \overrightarrow{\mathrm{rot}(\vec{H})} d\vec{s} = \oint_\delta \vec{H} d\vec{l} = \varepsilon \frac{\partial}{\partial t} \iint_S \vec{E} d\vec{s} + \sigma \iint_S \vec{E} d\vec{s} \qquad [2.41]$$

When one uses these results over the contour defined by the Yee cell (as shown in Figure 2.12), the circulation of the E field along the contour cannot consider the electric field being constant in the YEE cell (as it is in a regular FDTD cell).

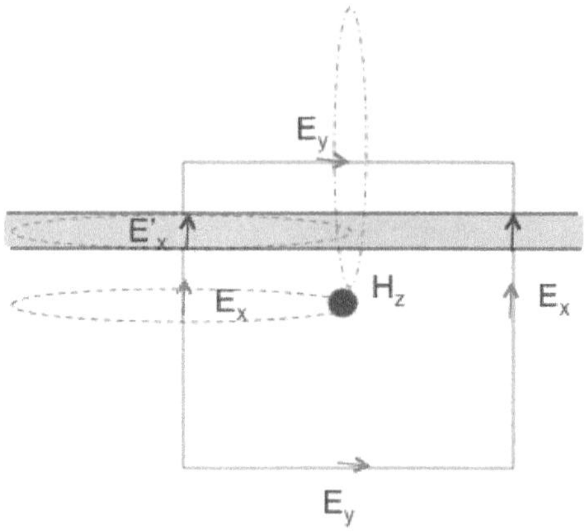

Figure 2.12. *Thin layer in an FDTD cell*

2.2.5. *Power and impedance in FDTD*

2.2.5.1. *Current, voltage and impedance in FDTD*

2.2.5.1.1. Current and voltage

The currents (I) and voltage (V) do not exist by themselves in the FDTD scheme. These quantities have to be accessed via the electric and magnetic fields.

The current is linked to the magnetic field [2.42] and can be seen as the sum of two components: the displacement current I_d and the conduction current I_c. The calculation of the circulation of the H field along a path δ surrounding a surface S (see Figure 2.13) gives:

$$I = \oint_{\delta} \vec{H}d\vec{l} = I_d + I_c = \varepsilon \frac{\partial}{\partial t} \iint_S \vec{E}d\vec{s} + \sigma \iint_S \vec{E}d\vec{s} \qquad [2.42]$$

Assuming, as shown in Figure 2.13, a uniform grid with Δ as spatial grid step and dt as time step, the conduction current (flowing in the conductor) is given by [2.43].

$$I_c = \sum \sum H_{i,j}^{n} \Delta - \varepsilon \Delta^2 \frac{\left[E_{\substack{vertical \\ i'}}^{n} - E_{\substack{verical \\ i'}}^{n-1} \right]}{dt} \qquad [2.43]$$

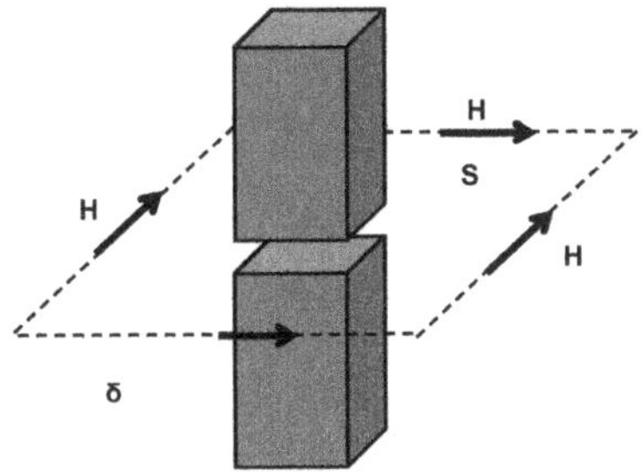

Figure 2.13. *Calculation of I through the circulation of H*

If the conductor is crossing the surface S and if the contour δ is close to the conductor, then the displacement current can be negligible and the conduction current is equal to the circulation of H. In all the cases, the current value is sampled at "H" time (i.e. with a dt/2 time difference with the "E" time).

The calculation of V is linked to the circulation of E along a path [2.44] that is less tricky than the conduction current assessment.

$$V = \int_L \vec{E}d\vec{l} \qquad [2.44]$$

Consider Figure 2.14, the voltage in the gap is the circulation of E in the gap; in this case and still considering a uniform grid with Δ as spatial grid step, $V = E_z\Delta$.

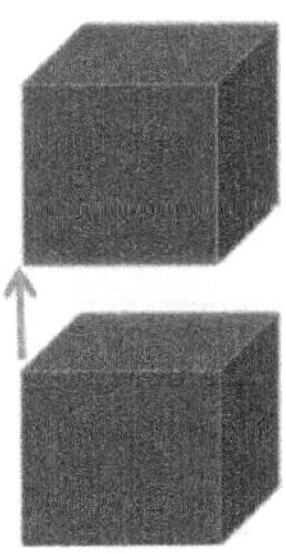

Figure 2.14. *Calculation of V through the circulation of E*

There are several methods that can be used within FDTD to inject energy within a system able to radiate [TAF 95, COS 09]. Among these methods, the simplest one is to force the E field value in the gap at each time step as shown in Figure 2.15.

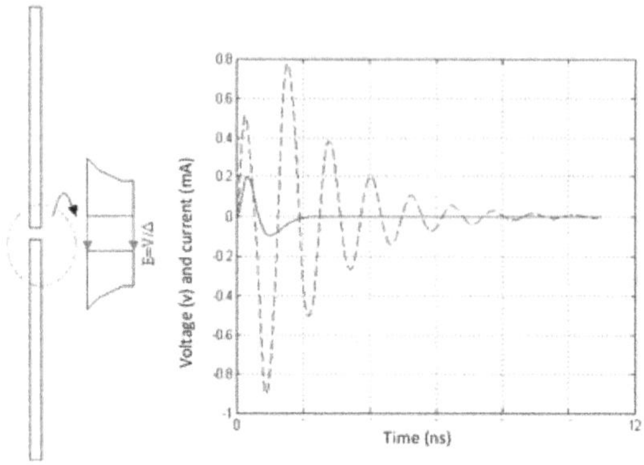

Figure 2.15. *Example of signal delivered in the GAP*

It is well known that the spectral occupancy of a signal is linked to its time variations. As shown in Figure 2.16, the sine has, as expected, a very narrow band but the steady state requires long computation duration. A good compromise seems to be a "gaussine" (mixture of sine and Gaussian).

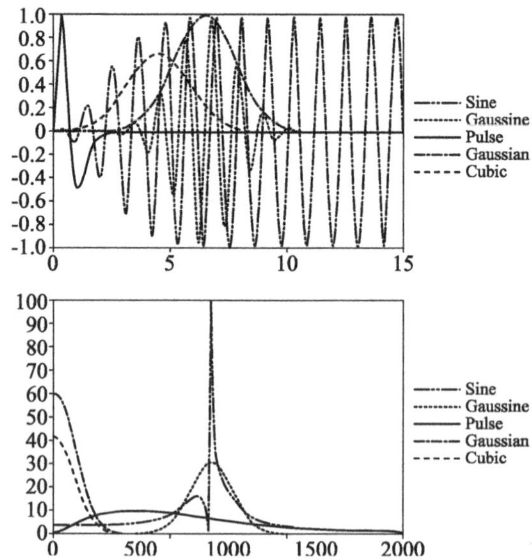

Figure 2.16. *Example of time and frequency pattern of input signals*

2.2.5.1.2. Impedance

The impedance is given by the ratio of tension (V) and current (I) in the frequency domain [2.45]

$$Z(f) = {}^{V(f)}\!\big/_{I(f)} \qquad [2.45]$$

As pointed out in section 2.2.5.1, in the FDTD, I and V are calculated at different time steps. As a consequence, if I and V are calculated through a fast Fourier transformation (FFT) of data coming from FDTD, then a coefficient taking into account the time difference has to be applied to the impedance ($e^{-j2\pi f\frac{dt}{2}}$). As an example, Figure 2.17 shows the dipole impedance assessment with FDTD.

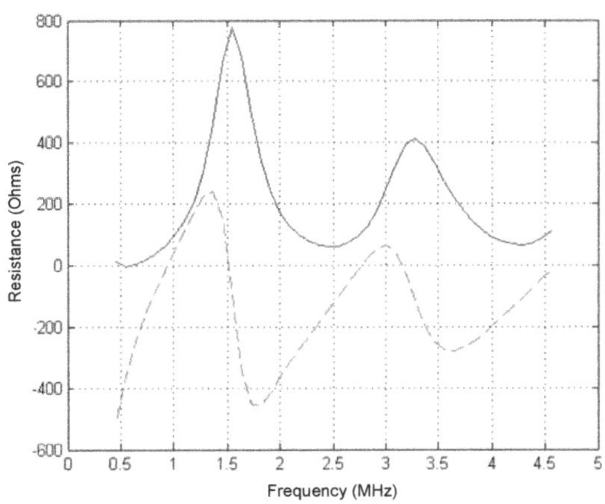

Figure 2.17. *Dipole impedance assessment with FDTD*

Knowing the current supplied to the antenna, the active and reactive powers supplied to the antenna can be derived using [2.46]:

$$P_{in} = I^*V = Z.\, I^*I \qquad [2.46]$$

2.2.5.2. *Power balance in FDTD*

Assuming a non-dispersive media, the combination of the Maxwell equations in the frequency and complex domain leads to [2.47]:

$$-\frac{1}{2}\overrightarrow{J_{in}^*}\vec{E} = \mathrm{div}\left(\frac{1}{2}\vec{E}\Lambda\overrightarrow{H^*}\right) + \sigma\frac{|E^2|}{2} + j\,2\omega\left[\mu\frac{|H^2|}{4} - \varepsilon\frac{|E^2|}{4}\right] \qquad [2.47]$$

where E and H are the electric and magnetic fields and J_{in}^{*} the conjugate of the current supplied to the sources in the volume *V*. The integration of [2.47] over a volume V surrounded by surface Ω shows that the power P_{in} supplied to the sources in the volume *V* is equal to the sum of the radiated and absorbed powers and average power stored in the electric and magnetic fields.

$$P_{in} = P_{rad} + P_{abs} + j\,2\omega(W_m - W_e) \qquad [2.48]$$

With the following definition:

$$P_{in} = -\frac{1}{2}\iiint_V \vec{J_{in}^{*}}\vec{E}\,dv = -\frac{1}{2}\iiint_V Re\left[\vec{J_{in}^{*}}\vec{E}\right]dv - j\,\frac{1}{2}\iiint_V Im\left[\vec{J_{in}^{*}}\vec{E}\right] \qquad [2.49]$$

$$P_{rad} = \frac{1}{2}\iint_\Omega \vec{E}\Lambda\vec{H^{*}}\,ds = \frac{1}{2}\iint_\Omega Re\left[\vec{E}\Lambda\vec{H^{*}}\right]ds + j\frac{1}{2}\iint_\Omega Im\left[\vec{E}\Lambda\vec{H^{*}}\right]ds \qquad [2.50]$$

$$P_{abs} = \frac{1}{2}\iiint_V \sigma|E^2|\,dv \qquad [2.51]$$

$$W_m = \iiint_V \mu\frac{|H^2|}{4}\,dv \text{ and } W_e = \iiint_V \varepsilon\frac{|E^2|}{4}dv \qquad [2.52]$$

Equation [2.49] provides the power supplied to the sources. By separating the real and imaginary parts, we obtain the active mean and reactive power [2.53] supplied by all the sources within *V* that can be linked to the impedance (section 2.2.5.1.2).

$$P_{In}^{active} = \iiint_V Re\left[\vec{J_{In}^{*}}\,\vec{E}\right]dv \quad \text{and} \quad P_{In}^{reactive} = -j\,\frac{1}{2}\iiint_V Im\left[\vec{J_{In}^{*}}\,\vec{E}\right] \qquad [2.53]$$

Equation [2.50] provides the power radiated that is equal to the flux of the Poynting vector through the surface Ω surrounding the volume V.

Equation [2.51] gives the absorbed power in the media. Dividing this P_{abs} by the mass in the volume V is providing the averaged Specific Absorption Rate (SAR) in the volume and the local SAR [2.55] as defined in the section 1.2.1.

$$\frac{P_{abs}}{M_{mass}} = \frac{\frac{1}{2}\iiint_V \sigma|E^2|dv}{\iiint_V \rho dv} = \frac{1}{V}\iiint_V \frac{\sigma|E^2|}{2\rho}dv = \frac{1}{V}\iiint_V SAR\,dv \qquad [2.54]$$

$$SAR = \frac{\sigma|E^2|}{2\rho} \qquad [2.55]$$

2.2.6. *FDTD and the Huygens box*

2.2.6.1. *Equivalence principle*

2.2.6.1.1. Regular case (non-crossing material)

In the case of a source far from the object under analysis (e.g. a person exposed to a base station far away), it is obviously quite impossible to model the source and the person together and compute this configuration with FDTD. In such a case, the equivalent principle [REN 00, MER 80, HOL 83] can be used, as illustrated in Figure 2.1, to take into account the field emitted by the RF without the effort of modeling it.

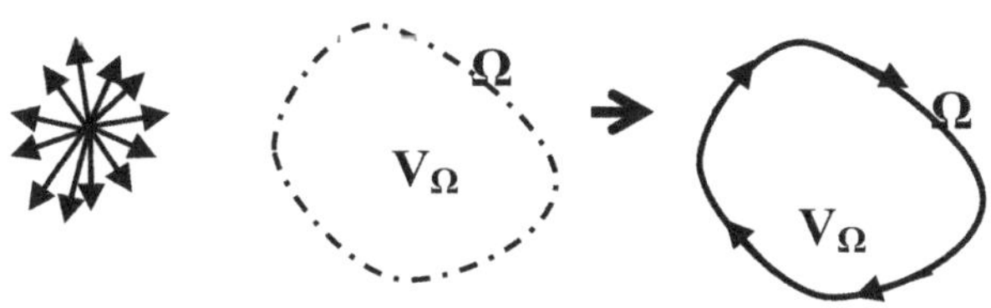

Figure 2.18. *Equivalent principle*

According to the equivalent principle, the assessment of the field induced in a volume V_Ω, limited by a surface Ω by a source located out of this volume can be carried out using equivalent currents, substituted into the original source and located on surface Ω. These currents allow having the E and H fields equal to those induced by the source in the V_Ω and 0 outside.

Let us consider $\{E_i, H_i\}$ the fields induced by the source and the Heaviside distribution U_{V_Ω} defined by [2.56].

$$U_{V_\Omega}(M)=1 \text{ if } M \in V_\Omega \text{ and } 0 \text{ if } M \notin V_\Omega \qquad [2.56]$$

Let us now consider the electric and magnetic fields weighted by this U_{V_Ω} [2.57], the electric and magnetic fields are those induced by the source in V_Ω and 0 outside.

$$\vec{E}(M) = U_{V_\Omega}(M).\vec{E_i}(M) \text{ and } \vec{H}(M) = U_{V_\Omega}(M).\vec{H_i}(M) \qquad [2.57]$$

In this equation, the EMF composed of $\{E_i, H_i\}$ complies with the Maxwell equations [2.1]. E and H have also to comply with the Maxwell equations; substituting [2.1] into [2.57] leads to [2.58]:

$$\overrightarrow{rot(\vec{E}(M,t)} = U_{V_\Omega}(M).\overrightarrow{rot(\vec{E_i}(M,t)} + \overrightarrow{grad(U_{V_\Omega}(M)} \wedge \vec{E_i}(M,t) \qquad [2.58]$$

The derivative of a Heaviside distribution is a Dirac distribution, [2.58] is therefore equivalent to [2.59]:

$$\overrightarrow{rot(\vec{E}(M,t)} = U_{V_\Omega}(M).\overrightarrow{rot(\vec{E_i}(M,t)} - \vec{n} \wedge \vec{E_i}(M,t).\delta_\Omega(M) \qquad [2.59]$$

The same approach can be taken with the H field. At the end, outside V_Ω the E and H field are null while they are equal to consider $\{E_i, H_i\}$ V_Ω that is what we were looking for. At the interface, J_Ω and M_Ω [2.60] are the equivalent current that have to be applied on the surface Ω to create the relevant electromagnetic field inside the volume.

$$M_\Omega = +\vec{n} \wedge \vec{E_i}(M,t).\delta_\Omega(M) \qquad [2.60]$$

$$J_\Omega = -\vec{n} \wedge \vec{H_i}(M,t).\delta_\Omega(M) \qquad [2.61]$$

Using this notation, the Maxwell equations are given by [2.62]:

$$\overrightarrow{rot(\vec{E})} = -\frac{\partial \mu \vec{H}}{\partial t} - \overrightarrow{M_\Omega} \text{ and } \overrightarrow{rot(\vec{H})} = \frac{\partial \varepsilon \vec{E}}{\partial t} + \sigma \vec{E} + \overrightarrow{J_\Omega} \qquad [2.62]$$

2.2.6.1.2. Crossing material

The previous developments have considered that the surface Ω was dividing the space in two parts. On the one hand the objects located in the volume V_Ω and on the other hand the sources that are located out of this volume V_Ω. Possible crossing material was not considered.

In some configurations, as shown in Figure 2.19, the whole material, in this case a wire, is not in the volume V_Ω and some material is crossing the surface. Such a case can occur with a small helix wire antenna connected to a phone box.

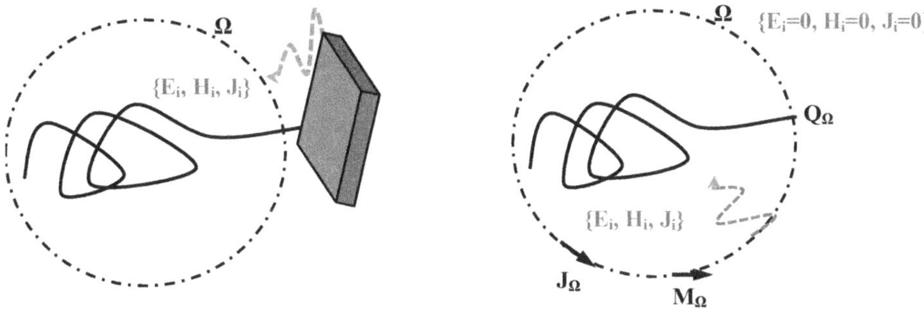

Figure 2.19. *Equivalent principle with crossing material*

In this case we need to use all the Maxwell equations. At the location M(x,y,z) and time t, the electric $\overrightarrow{E(M,t)}$ and magnetic $\overrightarrow{H(M,t)}$ fields radiated by the antenna in free space are governed by equations [2.1] and [2.2] but also by equations [2.63], [2.64] and [2.65] involving the charge density $\rho(M,t)$ and the current density $\overrightarrow{J(M,t)}$ and the continuity equation linking ρ and $\vec{J}$

$$\mathrm{div}\left(\varepsilon_0\overrightarrow{E(M,t)}\right) = \rho(M,t) \qquad [2.63]$$

$$\mathrm{div}\left(\mu_0\overrightarrow{H(M,t)}\right) = 0 \qquad [2.64]$$

$$\mathrm{div}\left(\overrightarrow{J(M,t)}\right) = -\frac{\partial\rho(M,t)}{\partial t} \qquad [2.65]$$

Following the same approach and notation as in section 2.2.6.1.1, let Ω be a surface enclosing a part of the antenna (Figure 2.19) in addition to the equations [2.57] we have also [2.66].

$$\overrightarrow{J(M,t)} = U_{V_\Omega}(M)\overrightarrow{J_1(M,t)} \qquad [2.66]$$

The combination of [2.65] and [2.66] creates a new relationship between $\rho(M,t)$ and $\overrightarrow{J(M,t)}$:

$$\mathrm{div}\left(\overrightarrow{J(M,t)}\right) = -\frac{\partial\rho(M,t)}{\partial t} - \left[-\vec{n}\overrightarrow{J_1(M,t)}\delta_\Omega\right] \qquad [2.67]$$

Thus, the EMF appears as radiated by the equivalent electric and magnetic currents J_Ω [2.60] and M_Ω [2.61] but also a localized charge density Q_Ω [2.68]:

$$Q_\Omega = \vec{n}\vec{J_1}(M,t).\delta_\Omega(M) \qquad [2.68]$$

2.2.6.2. *"Huygens box" implementation in FDTD*

As explained in the previous section, the objective is to add equivalent current, at the surface of a volume, that is representing the sources that are not modeled using voxel model. Figure 2.20 shows the "Huygens box" implementation in FDTD.

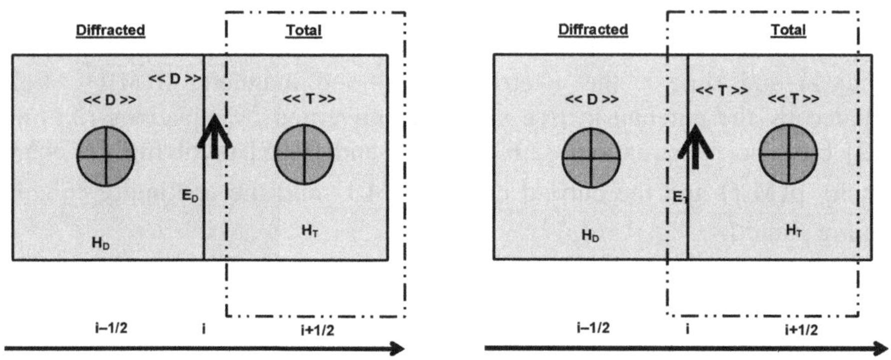

Figure 2.20. *Huygens box implementation in FDTD*

The Huygens box implementation in FDTD is not complex but can be cumbersome because of the index management. Some quantities have to be added or removed depending on the configuration; this process must be carried out carefully close to the edge or corner in order to avoid multiple addition or subtraction.

2.2.6.3. *Huygens box use for plane and spherical wave*

2.2.6.3.1. Plane waves

The Huygens box implementation in FDTD is quite easy in case of plane wave since the incident field can be expressed (using the usual notation,

$\{\omega, \vec{k}\}$, for the frequency and the propagation vector) in a close form (e.g. [2.69] for the E field):

$$\vec{E}(t, x, y, z) = \vec{E_0} e^{j2\pi ft - (jk_x x + jk_y y + jk_z z)} \quad [2.69]$$

This approach allows calculating the incident field value at the exact location of the field component in the cell.

$$E_x(n, i, j, k) = \vec{E_0} e^{j2\pi fndt - [jk_x\left(i-\frac{1}{2}\right)dx + jk_y jdy + jk_z kdz)} \quad [2.70]$$

It is important to point out that in equations [2.69] and [2.70], the vector $\vec{k}$ refers to the theoretical propagation in free space. For instance, in free space $\|\vec{k}\| = \frac{c}{f}$ with c being the light velocity in free space. As explained in section 2.2.2.2, the numerical velocity is not exactly the theoretical one, so the theoretical incident field that is planned to be added or removed according to sections 2.2.6.1 and 2.2.6.2 can differ from the value that needs to be added or removed because of different propagation time due to different velocities. This problem can be partially solved by replacing in equations such as [2.70] the numerical value of $\vec{k}$ that can be obtained numerically using [2.18]. This approach improves the result but does not eliminate all the problems, indeed the numerical velocity not only depends on the grid size but also on the angle of incidence.

2.2.6.3.2. Spherical waves

As explained previously, the equivalence principle is often used to avoid non-useful free space meshing; this method has proven its efficiency when the coupling between the source and the exposed object can be negligible. Most of the time, only planc wavcs are modeled. With the recent use of systems such as small cells that are quite close to users, the plane wave model is discussable. An efficient way to overcome this limit is to use the spherical waves expansion (SWE)

The EMF is often expressed as a plane wave expansion (as in the previous section) in the Cartesian coordinates. Since the spherical waves are orthogonal, EMF can be also expressed, in the spherical coordinates, as a SWE [HOL 83]. Let us consider r as the radius between the observation point and the sources, θ as the elevation angle φ the azimuth angle, let us also note λ as the wavelength in free space, k as the wave number given by

$^{2\pi}/_{\lambda}$ and η as the specific admittance. Using these notations the electric and magnetic fields (see Figure 2.21), $\{\vec{E}(r,\theta,\varphi), \vec{H}(r,\theta,\varphi)\}$, in the spherical coordinates can be expressed using the SWE given by [2.71] and [2.72]:

$$\vec{E}(r,\theta,\varphi) = \frac{k}{\sqrt{\eta}} \sum_{s=1}^{2} \sum_{n=1}^{N} \sum_{m=-n}^{n} Q_{smn} \vec{F}_{smn}(r,\theta,\varphi) \quad [2.71]$$

$$\vec{H}(r,\theta,\varphi) = -ik\sqrt{\eta} \sum_{s=1}^{2} \sum_{n=1}^{N} \sum_{m=-n}^{n} Q_{smn} \vec{F}_{3-s,m,n}(r,\theta,\varphi) \quad [2.72]$$

In this SWE, *N* is the number of modes, Q_{smn} and $\vec{F}_{smn}$ the coefficients and the spherical wave function of index s (TM or TE fields), order m and degree n. The spherical expansion should be composed of a finite number of modes, but a limited number is enough to have an accurate description of the field [JEN 04]. This limited number, *N*, of modes is enough. Even if, in theory, there is an infinite number of spherical modes, in practice, a finite number N of modes is to be chosen in order to be sufficient to correctly describe the field emitted by the antenna.

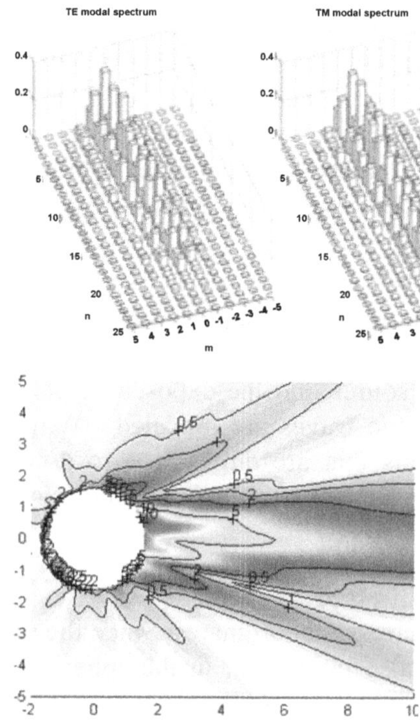

Figure 2.21. *Example optimal representation of the EM fields. For a color version of the figure, see www.iste.co.uk/wiart/radiofrequency.zip*

A method based on the SWE has been developed [HOL 83], to deduce the EMF emitted by an antenna in free space from spherical near-field measurements. As shown in Figure 2.21, the field emitted by antenna with complex radiated pattern can be represented with a limited number of modes with their complex weights.

2.2.7. *Near to far transformation and power radiated assessment*

2.2.7.1. *Near to far transformation*

The equivalent principle described in section 2.2.6.1 can be used to calculate the far field emitted by a source with a limited calculation. The electromagnetic fields emitted by sources located in a volume V surrounding by a surface Ω (see Figure 2.22) can be calculated by equivalent electric and magnetic surface currents J_Ω and M_Ω located at the surface Ω (a current that only flows tangential to the interface).

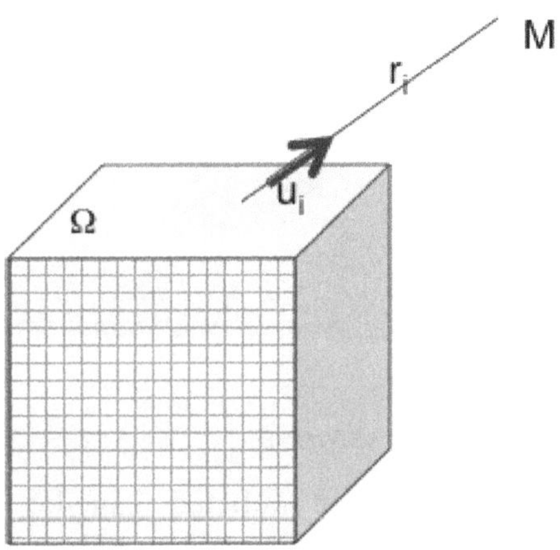

Figure 2.22. *Far field estimation*

J_Ω is the "usual" electric surface current and is given by [2.73]. M_Ω is the magnetic surface current (that does not exist in reality and is only useful in this mathematical representation) and is given by [2.74]:

$$\overrightarrow{J_\Omega}(r, f_0) = \vec{n}(r) \wedge \vec{E}(r, f_0) \qquad [2.73]$$

$$\overrightarrow{M_\Omega}(r, f_0) = \overrightarrow{-n(r)} \wedge \vec{H}(r, f_0) \qquad [2.74]$$

The electric field induced by these sources in the far field and in the direction $\vec{k}(\theta, \varphi)$ can be given by [2.75] and [2.76]:

$$E_\theta = \left[-\sqrt{\frac{\mu}{\varepsilon}} N_\theta(r, f_0) + L_\varphi(r, f_0)\right] \frac{\sqrt{\varepsilon\mu}}{2f_0} \frac{e^{j\vec{k}\vec{r}}}{|\vec{r}|} \quad [2.75]$$

$$E_\varphi = \left[-\sqrt{\frac{\mu}{\varepsilon}} N_\varphi(r, f_0) + L_\theta(r, f_0)\right] \frac{\sqrt{\varepsilon\mu}}{2f_0} \frac{e^{j\vec{k}\vec{r}}}{|\vec{r}|} \quad [2.76]$$

where $\{N_\theta, N_\varphi\}$ and $\{L_\theta, L_\varphi\}$ are derived from equations [2.77] and [2.78]:

$$N(r, f_0) = \mu \iint_\Omega \overrightarrow{J_\Omega(\vec{r'}, f_0)} e^{-j\vec{k}(\overrightarrow{r} - \vec{r'})} ds' \quad [2.77]$$

$$L(r, f_0) = \mu \iint_\Omega \overrightarrow{M_\Omega(\vec{r'}, f_0)} e^{-j\vec{k}(\overrightarrow{r} - \vec{r'}} ds' \quad [2.78]$$

Figure 2.23 shows an example of application with a mobile phone close to the head.

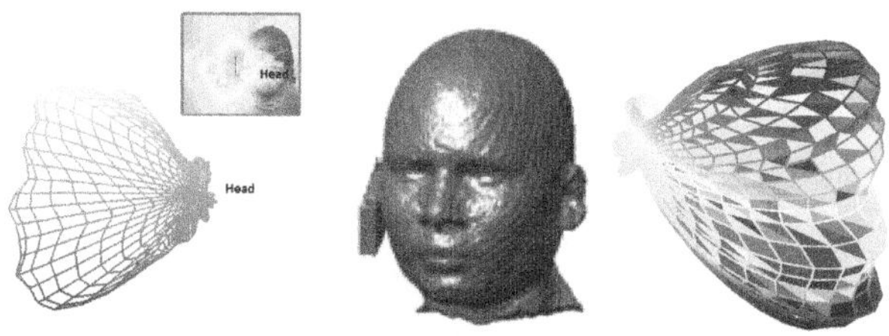

Figure 2.23. *Example of near to far application. For a color version of the figure, see www.iste.co.uk/wiart/radiofrequency.zip*

2.2.7.2. *Power radiated assessment*

The assessment of the power radiated can be performed by two approaches. The first is based on the formula [2.48]; in this case the radiated power is derived from the input power (Pin) and the absorbed power (Pabs). The second approach is based on the calculation of the flux of the Poynting vector through a surface Ω surrounding the radiating object. If the surface is in the far field (then the surface of a sphere can be used) the Poynting vector can be calculated using the formula described in section 2.2.7.1. If the NF-FF formulas have not been implemented, then the power radiated can also be assessed using flux of the Poynting vector through the surface Ω [2.50] surrounding, as shown in Figure 2.22, a cubic volume V. To perform the integration of the Poynting vector, the E and H have to be estimated in the frequency domain and at the same location.

2.3. FDTD and human exposure assessment

2.3.1. *SAR estimation using FDTD*

The SAR (specific absorption rate, defined in section 1.2.1, equation [1.4], SAR = $(\frac{\sigma E^2}{2\rho})$) assessment in a given voxel not only requires knowing the dielectric property of the media composing the cell but also the electric field strength in the cell. The FDTD that is using the Yee cell (Figure 2.1) and the leap-frog provides the E field components located on the edge of the cell. As shown in Figure 2.24, the calculation of the E field strength involved in the SAR calculation will require us to use field components located on the edge of the Yee cell.

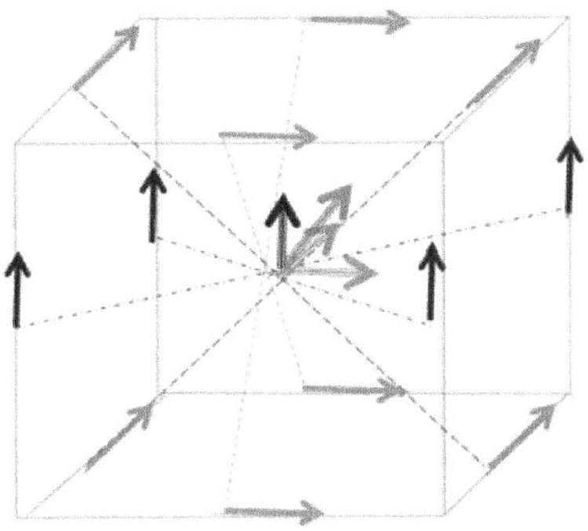

Figure 2.24. *Electric field strength estimation in voxel*

The dielectric properties of human tissue depends on frequency. As a consequence, the E field strength involved in the SAR estimation is the E field strength assessed at a given frequency while the E field components in the FDTD are time dependent with an E field strength, $E(n\,\Delta\,t) = \|E(n\,\Delta\,t)\|$, given by [2.79]:

$$E_{i,j,k}(n\Delta t) = E(i\Delta x, j\Delta y, k\Delta z, t) = \sqrt{\left(E_{x_{i,j,k}}(n\Delta t)\right)^2 + \left(E_{y_{i,j,k}}(n\Delta t)\right)^2 + \left(E_{z_{i,j,k}}(n\Delta t)\right)^2} \qquad [2.79]$$

With simulations performed at a single frequency (e.g. with a sine function), the E field strength is easily extractable. If these simulations involve signals having large frequency bands, the assessment of the field strength at a given frequency needs specific tools such as a discrete fast Fourier transform (DFFT). This DFFT has to be performed [2.80] using for all the $\{i, j, k\}$ of interest the N value of E field components in the FDTD calculated at $n\,\Delta\,t$ $(0 \leq n \leq N)$.

$$\mathrm{DFFT}\{E_{i,j,k}(n\Delta t)\} = \mathrm{DFFT}\left\{\sqrt{\left(E_{x_{i,j,k}}(n\Delta t)\right)^2 + \left(E_{y_{i,j,k}}(n\Delta t)\right)^2 + \left(E_{z_{i,j,k}}(n\Delta t)\right)^2}\right\} \quad [2.80]$$

This estimation requires additional calculations and memory; these resources are not necessarily available. Because of that, the E field strength in a voxel {i,j,k} is often approximated using [2.81].

$$E(n\Delta t) \approx \left[\sqrt{\left(\mathrm{FFT}\left[E_{x,_{i,j,k}}(t)\right]\right)^2 + \left(\mathrm{FFT}\left[E_{y,_{i,j,k}}(t)\right]\right)^2 \left(\mathrm{FFT}\left[E_{z\ i,j,k}(t)\right]\right)^2}\right] \quad [2.81]$$

In doing this, it is important to keep in mind that such approximation induces uncertainty since the DFFT of the field strength is not equal to the root mean square of the DFFT of the components [2.82].

$$\mathrm{DFFT}[E(t)] \neq \left[\sqrt{\left(\mathrm{DFFT}\left[E_{x,_{i,j,k}}(t)\right]\right)^2 + \left(\mathrm{DFFT}\left[E_{y,_{i,j,k}}(t)\right]\right)^2 + \left(\mathrm{DFFT}\left[E_{z\ i,j,k}(t)\right]\right)^2}\right] \quad [2.82]$$

Figure 2.25 shows the FDTD calculations of the electric field strength and the SAR induced by a mobile operating at 900 Hz. We can observe that the mobile's model is a rough modeling of an old type of phone composed of a box and an extractable antenna.

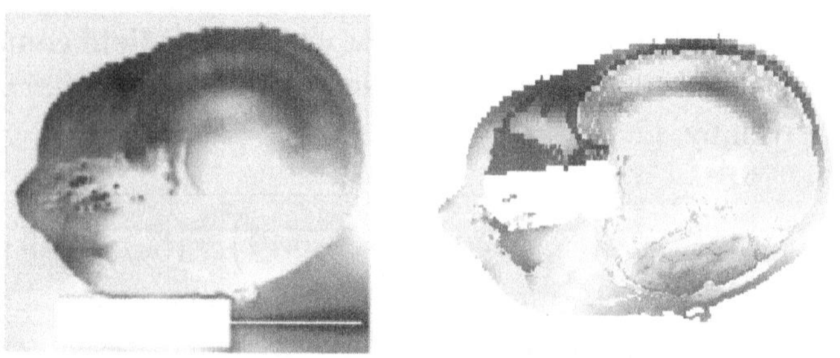

Figure 2.25. *Electric field (left) and SAR (right) induced in the head by a handset operating at 900 MHz*

2.3.2. *Anatomical numerical human models*

2.3.2.1. *Introduction*

The numerical (or computational) human models can be classified into four main categories. The first one, the oldest, is composed of "mathematical" models [XU 10, FIS 66, HWA 76, BAR 79, CRI 80, LEE 34]. In this case, the models are composed of spheres, cylinders, cones, ellipsoids and elliptical cylinders. These phantoms were mainly dedicated to ionizing studies; they were "stylized" phantoms composed of simplistic volumes (e.g. spheres for the head, cylinders for the trunk, arms and legs) that are easy to scale but of limited interest for RF exposure because in this frequency domain the organ shapes play important roles. The second category is composed of models based on images obtained using computed tomography (CT) performed during medical examinations [ZAN 35, PET 36]. A CT scan induces a significant exposure to ionizing radiations; consequently, the CT images of patients focus on specific organs so the whole-body models built with these images are composed of different set of images. The third category groups the models based on CT and photographic image of slices from donated cadavers. National projects from United States, Korea and China have supported this "visible human" approach[2,3] [ZHA 25, PAR 05, XU 00][4]. These models are anatomically correct with a very good resolution but, for ethical reasons, only a few models exist.

The last category is composed of models based on magnetic resonance imaging (MRI). In this category, the images were obtained during medical examinations or especially for this purpose [KIM 08]. The important development and increasing use of medical imaging, and the high resolution that allows MRI have led to the development of 3D human model voxels. Each voxel is defined so that it contains a uniform medium and is assigned an index that identifies it as belonging to a particular organ or tissue.

Even though large efforts have been carried out, only a few 3D and heterogeneous numerical head models or those of whole-body humans, having millimeter resolution, exist worldwide. This is due to the large

2 http://www.nlm.nih.gov/research/visible/visible_human.html.
3 http://vkh3.kisti.re.kr/.
4 http://visiblehuman.epfl.ch.

numbers of contiguous images that are needed to build a human model but also because of the important works that are required to identify the tissues (a process known as segmentation) and build the voxel or surface models.

2.3.2.2. *Adult models*

As explained in section 2.3.2.1, only few heterogeneous numerical human models exit because of the important works required to build such models. The first "anatomical" model was "Blockman" [GAN 82] composed of 180 cells of various sizes arranged to best fit the contour of a man (see Figure 2.26) but the resolution of "Blockman" and the internal organs' description are not really compatible with the frequency used in wireless communication systems.

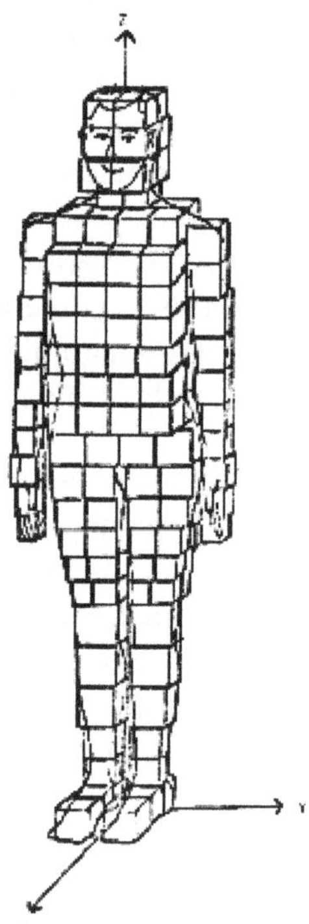

Figure 2.26. *Blockman*

In the RF domain, most of the numerical models of adults, anatomically correct and heterogeneous, that are used nowadays are based on photographic images, CT and MRI. As explained in section 2.3.2.1, only a few human adult models exit, most of them are based on MRI data and few are based on invasive investigation such as visible human. The objective of this section is not to provide an exhaustive description of all the existing models but to provide information on the most often used models. In the United States, two voxel human models have been developed. The first one, often known as "Zubal" [ZUB 94] has a resolution of $4 \times 4 \times 4$ mm^3; the second one is the well-known "visible human" [ACK 95] having a millimeter resolution. In the United Kingdom, two models, a male known as "Norman" and a female known as "Naomi", based on MRI images, have been developed [DIM 97, DIM 05] with a spatial resolution of $2 \times 2 \times 2$ mm^3. In Japan, whole-body voxel models of a Japanese adult male known as "Taro" and female [NAG 04] known as "Hanako" have been also developed based in MRI. The models were constructed on the basis of data obtained on volunteers – a 22-year-old Japanese man (height 172.8 cm, weight 65.0 kg) and woman (160.0 cm, 53.0 kg) – representative of average Japanese. The models are composed of 50 different tissues and organs with a spatial resolution of $2 \times 2 \times 2$ mm^3. In Korea, two adult male models have been built – one based on MRI [LEE 45] and the other on photographic images [KIM 08]. In Europe, two adult models (a male known as Duke and a female known as Ella), part of the Virtual Family [CHR 10], have been developed. They are based on MRI, composed of more than 80 tissues and have millimeter resolution. Recently, in China, two adult models (a male and a female) have been developed [WU 11] with a resolution of $1 \times 1 \times 1$ mm^3 and for female and male 90 and 87 tissues/organs have been identified, respectively. These models have been adapted to be handled by commercial code. In this case, the name can be changed as Hugo for VH. Figure 2.27 shows these phantoms.

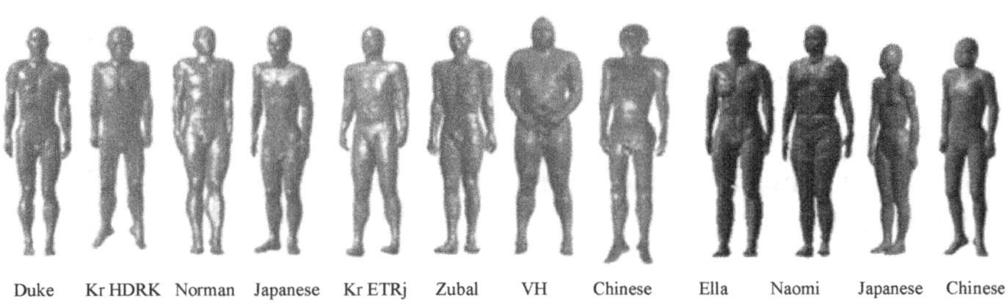

Figure 2.27. *Examples of 12 numerical models of adults (8 males on the left and 4 females on the right)*

Using some of these phantoms, studies have been carried [CON 08] out to assess the human exposure induced by a frontal plane wave from 20 MHz to 2.4 GHz (see section 2.4).

2.3.2.3. *Numerical child models*

Before the 1990s, most of the existing child models were developed for ionizing purpose and were mathematical computational models. With the progress in medical imaging and computer technology, different types of computational phantoms have appeared. On the one hand, there are the hybrid phantoms built for computational radiation dosimetry [LEE 10]. These models combine the flexibility of stylized phantoms (organ position and shape can be changed) and the anatomical realism of voxel phantoms that are not limited, as stylized phantoms are, by mathematical surface equations. On the other hand, there are the voxel phantoms based on MRI or CT that have the main advantage of being anatomically correct.

Because of the increasing use of RF wireless communication devices by children, several child head models have been developed. The first models have been created using a uniform downsizing of existing adult heads. However, a child head is not a reduced adult head [WIA 11, WIA 08]. For instance, the child's brain is growing quickly up to three years of age and is reaching 90% of the adult brain weight at five years of age [HUT 79]. The results performed with these kind of models have produced controversial results, the most eye-catching result is that from Gandhi's 1996 paper [GAN 96].

Other studies were performed to overcome these limitations and complement the existing models based on MRI [NAG 08, WAN 03, HAD 05, BRI 06]. In these studies, adult head models have been downscaled piecewise using a non-uniform downsizing taking into account the variation of the head shape with age.

As stated previously, the limits of these studies are linked to internal anatomy. Different tissues may have different growths. So as shown in Figure 2.28, external variations [FAR 94] cannot be representative of internal variations and any downsizing can lead to a wrong internal tissue distribution.

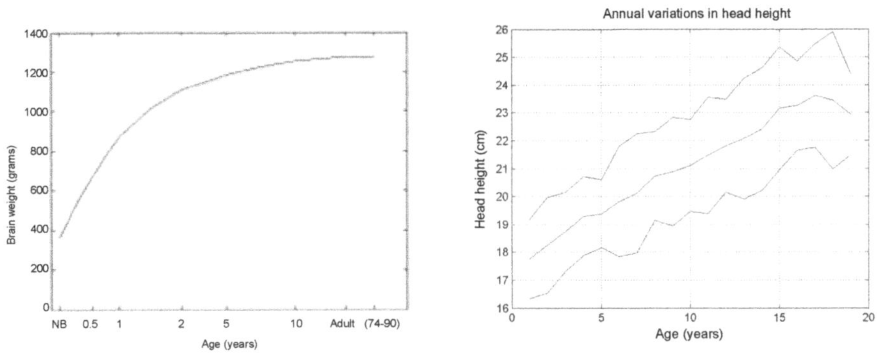

Figure 2.28. *Brain weight (left) and head height (right) versus age*

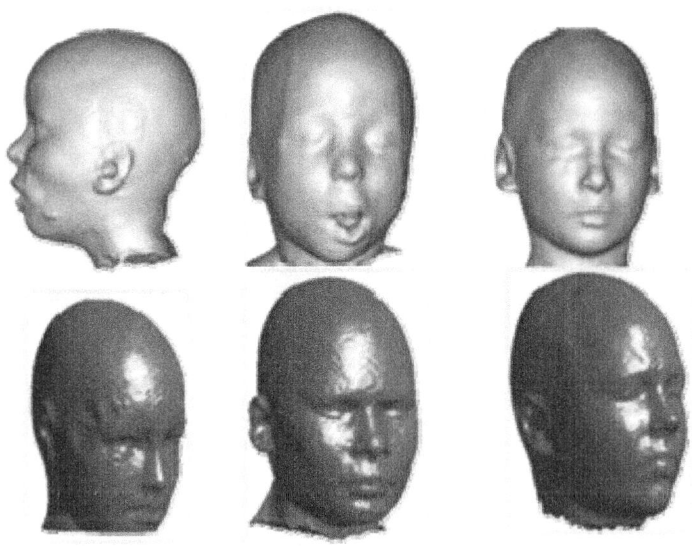

Figure 2.29. *Six child head models at 5, 6, 8, 9, 12 and 15 years of age [WIA 11]*

In spite of their limitations, these studies showed that the anatomy, the model of the handset and the position of the handset relative to the head have a large influence on the SAR induced in the tissues. Child head models based on MRI have therefore been developed [SCH 98, WIA 11, BUR 04]. Within the French National Research Agency (*Agence Nationale de la Recherche* (ANR)) project ADONIS [ADO 03] framework, several MRI datasets of children at different ages from three different French hospitals have been acquired with a spatial resolution of approximately 1 × 1 × 1.2 mm^3. They cover the whole head, thus allowing 3D segmentations directly in the 3D space. In this way, a good surface regularity of the tissues and structures is obtained [SCH 98]. Figure 2.30 shows six child head models at different ages (5, 6, 8, 9, 12 and 15 years old)

Because of the increasing use of wireless communication and because of the existing question on the whole-body SAR of children, several child body models have also been developed as shown in Figure 2.30. Among these models, we have Thelonius, Billie, Roberta, Dizzy, Eartha and Louis developed in the extended Virtual Family [GOS 14].

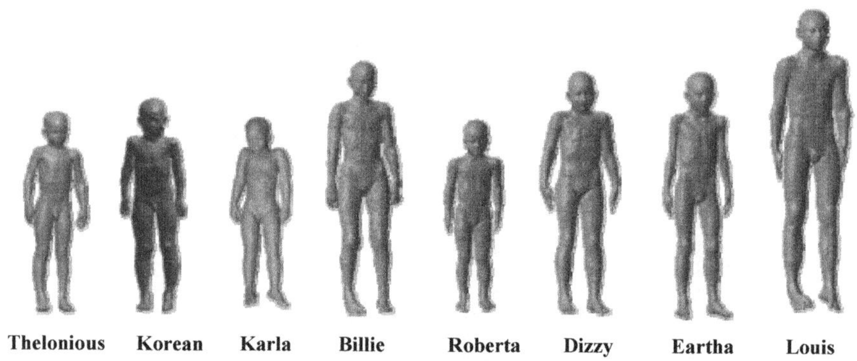

Figure 2.30. *Example of eight numerical models of children*

As shown in Figure 2.30, other child models have been developed such as the 7-year-old child in Korea [LEE 09] but these child models represent children older than 5 years while wireless communication system are used by very young children. A Common Sense Media research study published in 2013 in the United States shows, on the one hand, that 75% of American children have access to smartphones or tablets at home; on the other hand, this study also shows that 38% of children under 2 years of age play games or watch videos on these smart mobile.

Numerical models of very young children (from newborn to 3 years old) are very few and very often scaled models from older children or adult models [CON 08, LEE 07, CAS 13, HIR 08, PET 02]. These scaled models, even piecewise scaled, are facing difficulties [WIA 05, HAB 87]. To overcome them, a realistic 12-month-old numerical child model composed of 27 tissues with a resolution of $1 \times 1 \times 1$ mm^3 has been developed by the China Academy Telecom Research [LI 15] within the ANSES ACTE project[5] framework and compared with reference values from the Annals of the International Commission of Radiological Protection [ICR 89]. The young child model is shown in Figure 2.31.

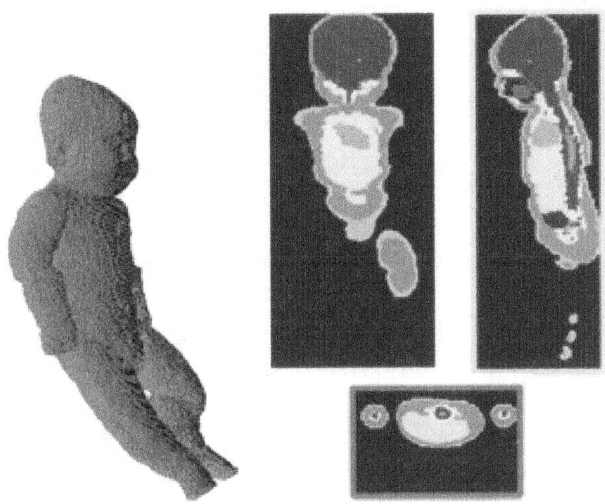

a) b)

Figure 2.31. *a) One-year-old child model. b) Axial, sagittal and coronal views of the model. For a color version of the figure, see www.iste.co.uk/wiart/radiofrequency.zip*

2.3.2.4. *Human model characteristics*

Even if the voxel body models have not been selected through a random process, there is a large variability of global parameters such as the body

5 http://whist.institut-telecom.fr/acte/.

mass index (BMI), height and mass (see Figure 2.32) characterizing the models described previously.

Analysis of the proportion of tissues in the body shows that the percentage of muscle is less variable than the bone's one (see Figure 2.33).

The analysis of the brain is of great interest for the children RF exposure analysis. As shown in Figures 2.32 and 2.33, the children's mass and height are smaller than those of the adults but the children's brain mass is similar to the adults while the proportion of brain (over the whole body) decreases (see Figure 2.34). Indeed, a child body cannot be modeled using a uniform downsizing.

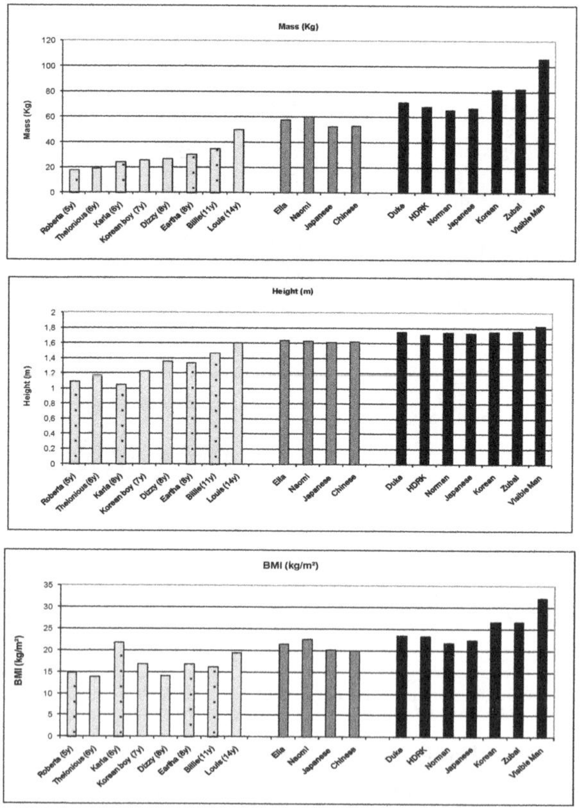

Figure 2.32. *BMI, height and mass*

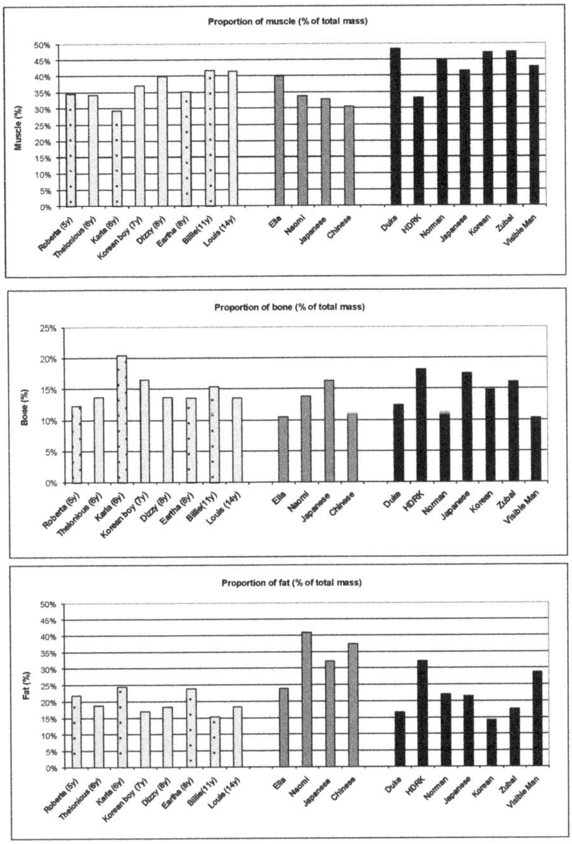

Figure 2.33. *Tissue proportions*

2.3.2.5. *Numerical fetus and pregnant woman models*

With the versatile use of wireless communication, the systems that are emitting RF can be used close to fetuses and pregnant women. In such contexts, WHO has recommended the study on the EMF dosimetry relating with fetuses as high-priority research topics. For ethical reasons, the fetus images are often acquired only for medical reasons and not for projects such as the RF dosimetry. The obstetrics images (Ultrasonic or MR) are therefore rarely whole-body images. As a consequence, full, anatomically correct, numerical models of heterogeneous pregnant women are rare; because of that, a hybrid approach is to insert utero-fetal units (UFUs) in a non-pregnant female model. In line with this approach, a few numerical heterogeneous pregnant female models have been developed [DIM 06, NAG 07]. But as stated in [VAR 14], these models are very specific to the fetus inserted while the position is variable as shown in Figure 2.35.

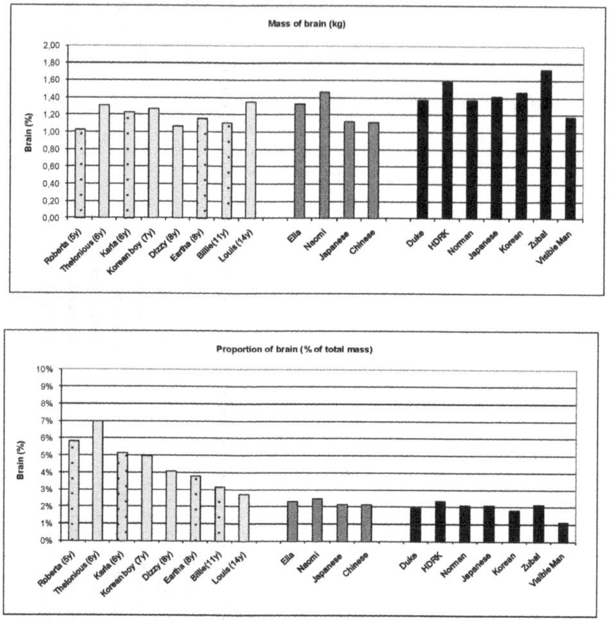

Figure 2.34. *Brain mass and proportions*

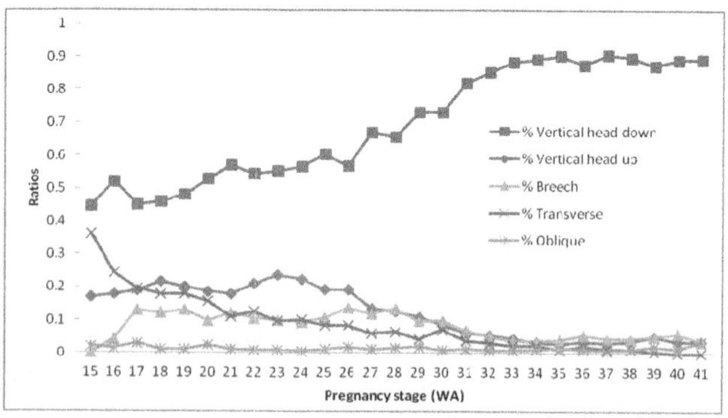

Figure 2.35. *Percentages of occurrences of various fetal positions during pregnancy at stages between 15 and 41 weeks of amenorrhea (WA). For a color version of the figure, see www.iste.co.uk/wiart/radiofrequency.zip*

To overcome this limitation, a deformable pregnant female model is needed. To achieve this objective, an initial French project, called Femonum [BIB 10], has been set up followed by an international project FETUS [VAR 14] funded by ANR in France and JST in Japan. A synthetic semi-homogeneous pregnant woman model within the range 8–32 weeks of amenorrhea (WA), using a fetus growth-modeling tool between 14 and 32 WA, has been developed [DAH 14]. From 8–13 WA, the UFUs were obtained from segmentation of ultrasound images [ANQ 09]. After 14 WA (within the range 14–32), the models are based on a combination of growth modeling and segmentation of MRI images, allowing the generation of UFUs.

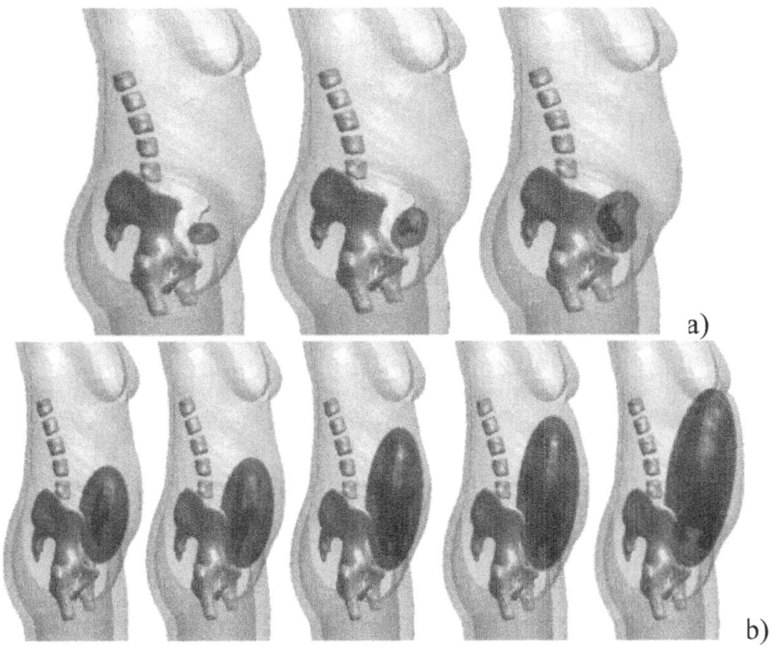

Figure 2.36. *Examples of developed pregnant female models obtained from segmentation of a) ultrasound images (three) and b) MRI (five on right)*

The 13 pregnant female models, having a millimeter resolution, developed within the FETUS and FENONUM projects are skin, the subcutaneous fat, the muscle, a pelvis, a UFU including the uterus, the uterine content, the fetal tissues (envelop, skull, brain and lung) and finally an homogeneous tissue replacing all the other organs and tissues inside. The tool developed in the fetus framework allows choosing the fat layer thickness of the synthetic female model [BIB 10].

The original non-pregnant female model weighs 75.5 kg for a height of 1.74 m, which corresponds to a BMI of 24.9. It contains 3.46 kg of subcutaneous fat. This weight stays constant during the pregnancy. The weight of each fetus model is coherent average fetal weight at the same pregnancy stages [VAL 89].

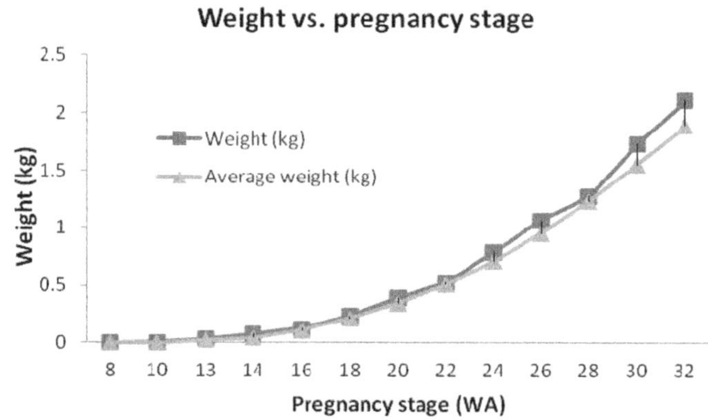

Figure 2.37. *Comparison of generated fetus weights and average fetal weights at the same pregnancy stages. For a color version of the figure, see www.iste.co.uk/wiart/radiofrequency.zip*

Since the medical images and the segmentation [ANQ 09] produced voxels, they are easy to use in the FDTD orthogonal grid but as explained previously the dielectric properties of the FDTD cell are highly variable. So as schematically shown in Figure 2.39, the FDTD scheme has to handle such variability.

2.3.3. *Heterogeneous and dispersive biological tissues*

2.3.3.1. *Heterogeneous tissues and FDTD*

The development of realistic human models will be addressed in other sections but in many cases the biological tissues are highly heterogeneous as shown in Figure 2.38.

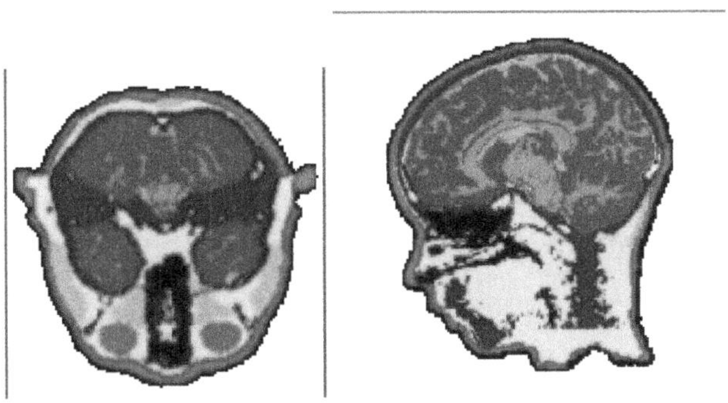

Figure 2.38. *Child head developed. For a color version of the figure, see: www.iste.co.uk/wiart/radiofrequency.zip*

In this case, the dielectric properties assigned to the FDTD cells are different from one cell to another one. As shown in Figure 2.1, the use of the well-known "Yee cell" leads to using in the numerical scheme E and H field components that are sampled on the edge or on the surface of the cell. In such a case, the dielectric properties involved in [2.21] are not those of one cell but possibly a combination of several dielectric properties.

To determine the value that has to be used, let us consider a non-dispersive, isotropic, heterogeneous and lossy dielectric media. The Maxwell equations are those given by [2.1] and [2.2]. A simple way is to decide that the dielectric properties of tissues used in the FDTD formulation are those of the cell. This means that $\{\varepsilon, \sigma\}$, which are used in [2.12], are $\{\varepsilon(i,j,k), \sigma(i,j,k)\}$ ignoring that the Ez is at the interface of possibly four different dielectrics.

To take into account the heterogeneity, let us now consider a surface S and the contour δ of this surface as described in Figure 2.40. E_z is tangential to the voxel so it can be considered as non-affected by the interface (i.e. E_z considered as constant over the surface S). The H field components (H_x and H_y) are perpendicular but since the media considered is equivalent to free space for the H field (no magnetic conductivity and free space permeability), then the H field components are also continuous.

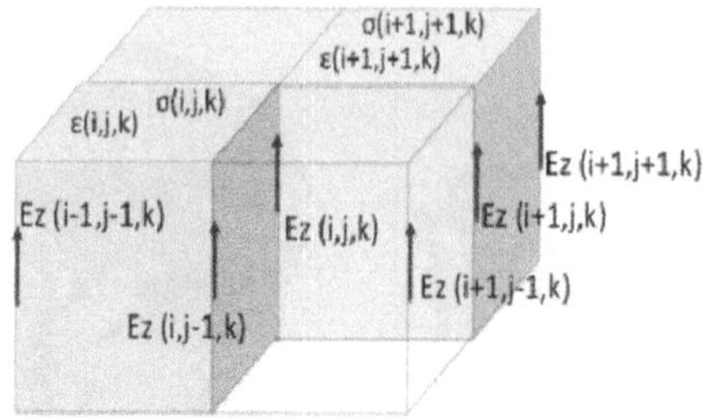

Figure 2.39. *Heterogeneous tissues modeled using FDTD cells*

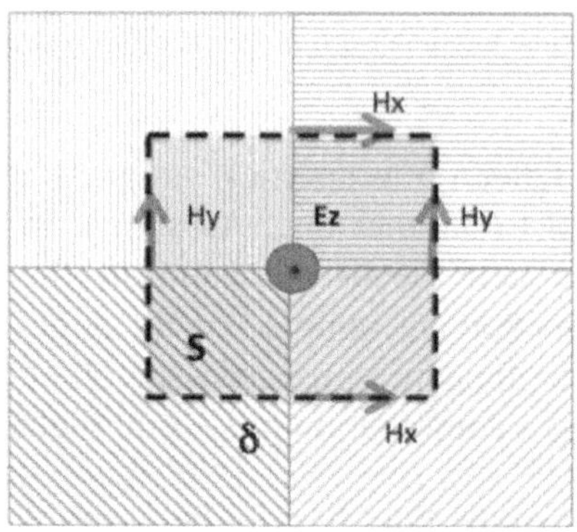

Figure 2.40. *Contour*

Taking into account the properties of E and H on the surface and along the contour, the integration of [2.2] over the surface S gives [2.83]:

$$\iint_S \overrightarrow{\mathrm{rot}(\vec{H})} d\vec{s} = \oint_\delta \vec{H} d\vec{l} = \frac{\partial E_z}{\partial t} \iint_S \varepsilon(x, y, z_0) d\vec{s} + E_z \iint_S \sigma(x, y, z_0) d\vec{s} \quad [2.83]$$

[2.83] provides equivalent permittivity $\varepsilon_{\mathrm{equivalent}}$ and conductivity $\sigma_{\mathrm{equivalent}}$ that are given by $\varepsilon_{\mathrm{equivalent}} = \iint_S \varepsilon(x, y, z) d\vec{s}$ and $\sigma_{\mathrm{equivalent}} = \iint_S \sigma(x, y, z) d\vec{s}$. With the FDTD notation (i.e. equation [2.7]) and for the z component of the E (i.e. E_z) field, the equivalent dielectric properties are expressed as:

$$\varepsilon_{Z\_\mathrm{equivalent}} = \frac{\varepsilon_{i,j,k} + \varepsilon_{i+1,j,k} + \varepsilon_{i,j,k} + \varepsilon_{i,j+1,k} + \varepsilon_{i+1,j+1,k}}{4} \quad [2.84]$$

$$\sigma_{Z\_\mathrm{equivalent}} = \frac{\sigma_{i,j,k} + \varepsilon_{i+1,j,k} + \sigma_{i,j,k} + \varepsilon_{i,j+1,k} + \sigma_{i+1,j+1,k}}{4} \quad [2.85]$$

2.3.3.2. *Dispersive and lossy biological tissues*

As stated previously, the human body is composed of various organs and tissues that are heterogeneous. In the RF domain, the properties of these tissues are isotropic but they are lossy and dispersive[6]. As an example, Figure 2.41 shows the variation of the skin and gray brain matter permittivity and conductivity with the frequency.

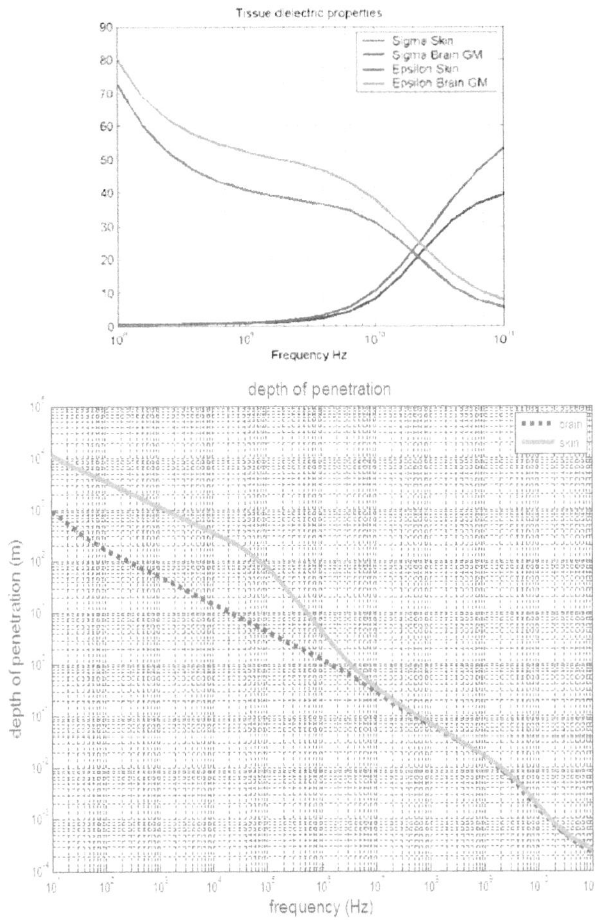

Figure 2.41. *Permittivity, conductivity and depth of penetration versus frequency for skin and brain gray matter. For a color version of the figure, see: www.iste.co.uk/wiart/radiofrequency.zip*

6 (See footnote 2).

Equations [2.1] and [2.2] consider the dielectric properties, for instance $\varepsilon(x, y, z)$ and $\sigma(x, y, z)$, as dependent on the location but these equations do not consider the dispersive properties. In such a case, the Maxwell equations are given by [2.86] and [2.87]:

$$\overrightarrow{\mathrm{rot}\left(\overrightarrow{E(M,t)}\right)} = -\frac{\partial\left(\overrightarrow{B(M,t)}\right)}{\partial t} \quad [2.86]$$

$$\overrightarrow{\mathrm{rot}\left(\overrightarrow{H(M,t)}\right)} = \frac{\partial\left(\overrightarrow{D(x,y,z,t)}\right)}{\partial t} + \sigma(M,t)\overrightarrow{E(M,t)} \quad [2.87]$$

With B sometimes defined as the magnetic induction and D the electric excitation defined by [2.88]:

$$\overrightarrow{B(M,t)} = \left(\mu(M,t) * \overrightarrow{B(M,t)}\right) \quad [2.88]$$

$$\overrightarrow{D(M,t)} = \left(\varepsilon(M,t) * \overrightarrow{E(x,y,z,t)}\right)$$

In these equations, the notation * represents the convolution as defined by [2.89]

$$\left(\varepsilon(M,t) * \overrightarrow{E(M,t)}\right) = \left\langle \varepsilon(M,t) \middle| \overrightarrow{E(M,t)} \right\rangle = \int_{-\infty}^{+\infty} \varepsilon(M,\tau) * \overrightarrow{E(M,t-\tau)}\, d\tau \quad [2.89]$$

In RF exposure assessment, the magnetic permeability is considered as equal to the free space ($\mu = \mu_0$) and not dispersive.

Figure 2.41 also shows that the dielectric properties of these tissues above 0.7 GHz can be considered as almost constant over a few hundred megahertz. Today, most of the time, except for the ultra-wide band (UWB) systems, RF communication systems use frequency bands lower than 100 MHz. In this case, for RF exposure assessment purposes, the dielectric properties can be considered as constant over the frequency band used by the communication system.

2.3.4. *FDTD sub-gridding and hybridization*

2.3.4.1. *Introduction*

The accuracy of the thin wire or layer can be limited and the "thin" methods cannot handle all the configurations. As described in section 2.2.4, even if Holland's approach is better adapted than Taflove's for processing tilted wires, these methods are not suitable in front of a small helical antenna as several phones had in the 1990s. Similarly, geometries having locally fine structures also challenge the usual FDTD. In this case, the use of fine grid requires large memory and long computational time. Nowadays, high-performance computation and GPU, for instance, can manage large problems and have postponed the need of local refinement. But if this improvement of the technology brought a palliative approach, it did not fundamentally solve this issue for the future. In the 2000s, computers were not as they are now and two approaches have been investigated to solve this problem: the sub-gridding and the hybrid approach.

2.3.4.2. *Sub-gridding*

A major drawback of the uniform FDTD is its difficulty in handling geometries that have locally fine structures. A dense mesh is, in this case, required all over the computational domain that can lead to unmanageable problems. For instance, the inner ear grid size must be close to 0.1 mm which in the case of a uniform grid induces extremely large problems. As described previously, a non-uniform grid can be used [WIA 98] to save memory but such an approach does not allow a local refinement of the grid. To alleviate this limitation, large efforts have been carried out in the 1990s to create sub-gridding [OKO 97, WON 03, PAS 07, CHA 99, BON 07]. The main advantage of the sub-gridding method is its ability to locally improve the field resolution, without modifying the rest of the computational domain. Several sub-gridding techniques have been proposed; some of these approaches were based on "interpolation schemes" in space and time with possibly an offset of the local grid [ANQ 09] (see Figure 2.42).

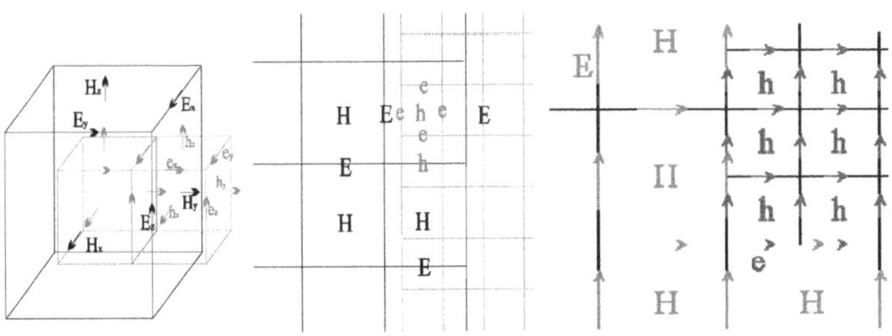

Figure 2.42. *Sub-grid schemes in space and time with an offset (left) and no offset (right) of the local grid. For a color version of the figure, see www.iste.co.uk/wiart/radiofrequency.zip*

Other methods were based on collocated fields [CHE 97] or Huygens boxes [BRE 06]. For any sub-gridding methods, obtaining a stable scheme is the most tricky objective to reach. Since the numerical velocity in the coarse grid is different from the one in the fine grid, instabilities can exist. Moreover, the errors introduced by the interpolation techniques can be summed up in the iterative FDTD time marching scheme and lead to other instabilities. Indeed, most of the sub-gridding techniques described in the literature are conditionally stable. To limit the error introduced at the interface, most of the sub-gridding algorithms described in the literature, the reduction factor is limited. To alleviate this limitation, nested local grids [PAS 07] have been investigated in order to increase the reduction factor.

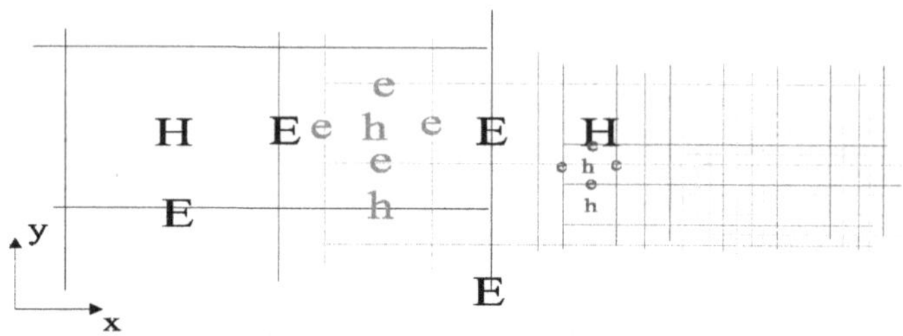

Figure 2.43. *Nested sub-gridding scheme. For a color version of the figure, see www.iste.co.uk/wiart/radiofrequency.zip*

The observed stability and accuracy of the nested mesh approach seems to be based on the small interpolation error and implicit weighting operations.

The progresses observed recently in computer technologies, memory and high-performance computation have postponed the need of local refinement but they did not eliminate the need for the future. Today, fewer efforts are carried out in this domain and the question of the stability is still open.

2.3.4.3. *Hybridation*

The regular orthogonal mesh of the FDTD is mainly the base of simplicity and efficiency of this method. This advantage, in counterpart, limits the flexibility to provide higher resolution locally or to conform to objects of arbitrary shapes. Fine resolution, even if costly from the memory and computational time point of view, can alleviate such a limit. Non-uniform FDTD, even if less accurate, can also partially reduce these limitations but they are not able to solve all the limits. Hybrid methods can be the optimal option to combine all the advantages of existing methods. Large efforts have been carried out in the 1990s and the 2000s to develop such hybrid methods, including the sub-gridding as it can be seen as a specific hybrid method since it combines two FDTD methods with different grid sizes.

2.3.4.3.1. FEM-FDTD

As explained previously, the main problem of the sub-gridding is the stability. Based on the use of a fine grid around critical areas within a coarse one, the main issue is related to exchange of information at the boundary between the two meshes, which renders a scheme stable or not. To avoid such a question, the FDTD sub-gridding scheme can be seen as a special case of a finite-element time domain (FETD) [BON 02, WON 03] since the classical FDTD Yee's scheme can be obtained from FETD [WON 95].

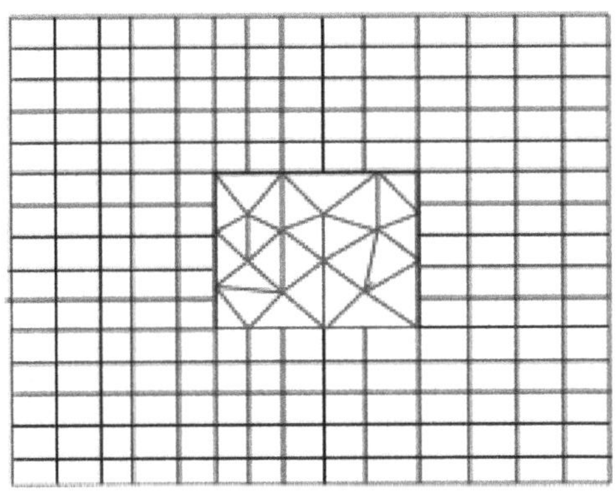

Figure 2.44. *Hybridization of FDTD and FETD*

2.3.4.3.2. MOMTD-FDTD

As described previously, the FDTD method is very efficient for large and heterogeneous problems but, because of the conformal mesh and of the stair case modeling, a major drawback of this method is its difficulty in managing thin wire structures having arbitrary orientations. Conversely, the MoM [HAR 87] and the method of moments in the time domain (MoMTD) [MIL 73, BRE 89] are known to be very efficient for modeling this kind of wire composed of perfect electric conductors (PECs). The MoM and MOMTD methods require a matrix inversion but at the instantaneous level, as shown in Figure 2.45, a wire segment interacts with itself and the neighbor segments. Therefore, the matrix involved in MoMTD is tri-diagonal that is quite easy to invert.

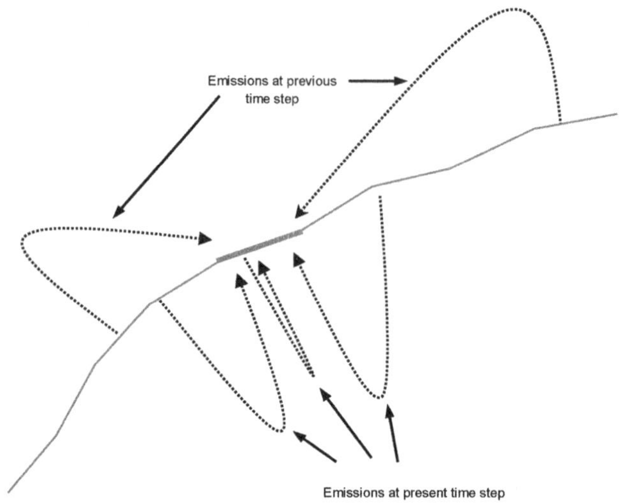

Figure 2.45. *EM time domain interactions of wire segment*

As MoM, the MoMTD has strong limitations with complex structures and is much less efficient than FDTD in this case. The combination of the advantages of FDTD and MoMTD [BRE 98] can overcome their limits. In this case, the idea is to use the equivalent principle (section 2.2.6.1) to transfer, at each time step, in the FDTD domain the EM field induced by the wire antenna and calculated using the MoMTD and to use the interpolation to assess on the wire the EM field calculated with FDTD (see Figure 2.46). Considering a surface Ω enclosing the wire antenna,the magnetic and electric currents at the surface Ω are calculated using the E and H fields (section 2.2.6.1) estimated with the MoMTD. To calculate the external variation, that is applied to the wire with the MoMTD method, there are two options. The first, applicable if the wire and object can be located in the FDTD computational domain as shown in Figure 2.46 (left), is the interpolation on the wire of the E field calculated by the FDTD at each time step.

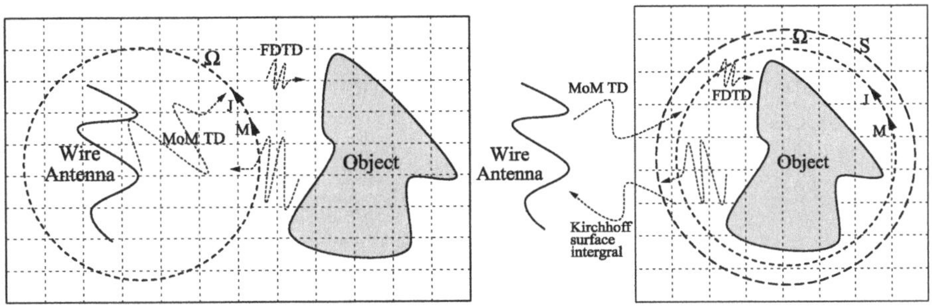

Figure 2.46. *MoMTD – FDTD with a wire located in (left) or out of (rigth) the FDTD computational domain*

The second approach that can be used if the wire is not in the FDTD computational domain (see Figure 2.46 (right)) is similar to a near field-to-near field (NF–NF) transformation.

Different NF–NF methods exist [OMA 97, SHL 95]; with the Kirchhoff representation, only three surface integrals have to be calculated while with the Stratton–Chu representation [STR 41] five integrals are required. According to the literature, the Kirchhoff representation therefore reduces the required memory storage volume by approximately 30% compared to a Stratton–Chu representation. Using the notation of Figure 2.47 and the Kirchhoff NF–NF transformation, the $\vec{E}(\vec{r},t)$ field at the observation point $\vec{r}$ and at the time t and using the $\vec{E}$ field on S at previous time is given by [2.90]:

$$\vec{E}(\vec{r},t) = \frac{1}{4\pi}\oint_S \vec{n}\left\{\frac{\vec{r}-\vec{r}\prime}{|\vec{r}-\vec{r}\prime|^3}\vec{E}\left(\vec{r}',t\right) + \frac{\vec{r}-\vec{r}\prime}{C|\vec{r}-\vec{r}\prime|^3}\frac{\partial\,\vec{E}(\vec{r}\prime,t\prime)}{dt'} + \frac{\vec{r}-\vec{r}\prime}{|\vec{r}-\vec{r}\prime|}\vec{\nabla}\vec{E}\left(\vec{r}',t\right)\right\}ds \qquad [2.90]$$

where $\vec{r}'$ is the vector coordinate of the source point (Figure 2.47), $\vec{n}$ the outward pointing normal to the closed surface S and t' the retarded time $t' = t - \frac{|\vec{r}-\vec{r}\prime|}{c}$.

Both approaches (interpolation and NF–NF) of the hybridation have been implemented and compared [LAU 04]. With the NF–NF transformation, the total required memory storage and the computation time depend on the number of segments used to model the antenna. But in the case of NF–NF transformation, the total storage is also a function of the number of cells that subdivide the surface S. Thus, this NF–NF approach is highly costly in memory storage and expensive in computation time. Conversely, the spatial interpolation method is simple, can be implemented rapidly and does not require unmanageable memory and computation time if the antenna is close to the object.

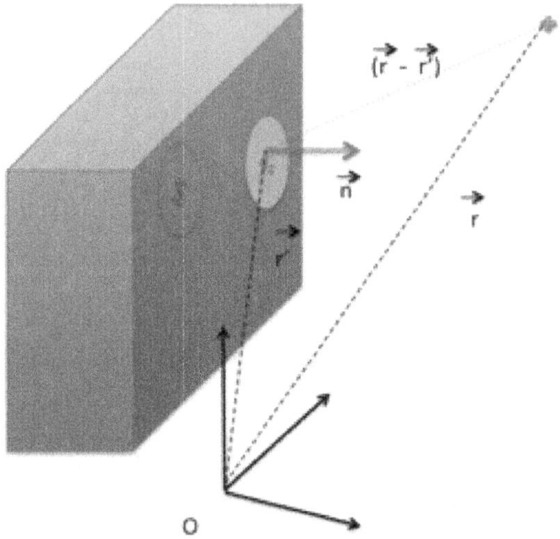

Figure 2.47. *Notation used to calculate the near-field-to-near field transformation*

To carry out an SAR calculation to assess the exposure induced by a mobile phone composed of a wire antenna, the interpolation approach can be used since the mobile phone does not increase a lot the computational domain.

At this point, it is important to point out that for both approaches the time step used by FDTD-MoM-TD must comply with both stability criteria that have been studied [YEE 66, LAU 00] using

$$\Delta t_{hybrid} = min\{\Delta t_{FDTD}, \Delta t_{MoMTD}\} \quad [2.91]$$

With the MoM-TD, the wire is, as shown in Figure 2.45, modeled using straight wire segments having ΔS length. In this case, the stability requires that ΔS is few time larger that the wire radius and for causality reason that $dt < \frac{\Delta S}{c}$. With the FDTD, the time step is linked to the grid step and in bio-electromagnetism often close and below a tenth of wavelength. Is this case, the FDTD time step is leading the simulations. As a consequence, to comply with the causality principle, ΔS is small and can lead to a large number of wire segments and because of that can induce large computation time (even the simple matrix inversion requires time). This can greatly reduce the value of the method and is a fundamental limit of the MoMTD-FDTD hybrid method.

Figure 2.48 illustrates the use of such hybrid method [STR 41] with a vertical helical antenna operating at 4.5 GHz and located in the proximity of a PEC ground plane at a distance of 15 mm.

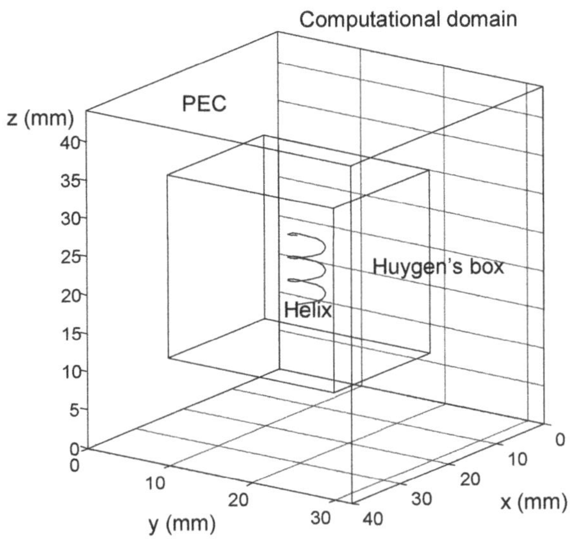

Figure 2.48. *Wire helix close to PEC*

The pitch is 3 mm, the total helix height is 9 mm and there are three turns. The helix diameter and wire diameter are, respectively, 4 and 0.6 mm. The antenna model for the MoMTD is composed of 42 segments and excited at its second segment. It is not only important to accurately represent the helical antenna, but also, as explained previously, to ensure that the MoMTD time step is compatible with the FDTD one. In the FDTD, a cell size of 2 mm has been chosen to compare to the minimum of 0.6 mm that should have been used to model the wire. The results obtained via the hybrid scheme are compared with those calculated by the method of images used in conjunction with the MoMTD alone. The field strength value has been analyzed for both approaches at a point located at 2 mm from the ground plane. As shown in Figure 2.49, the hybrid approach provides good results (average relative error less than 3%).

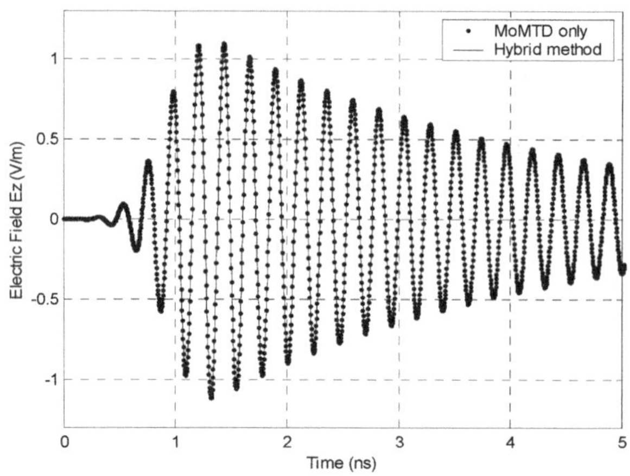

Figure 2.49. *Comparison of simulation carried with MoMTD + images versus MoMTD-FDTD for a helix antenna close to PEC*

At this stage, the first result we can draw is that the method is accurate but requires a very large computation time that is not necessarily compatible with the objectives of the numerical dosimetry and partly explains the very marginal use of this hybrid method.

Another limitation of the above approach is related to the connection of the wire antenna to the transmitter (e.g. body of the phone). In this case, unlike Figure 2.46, it is not possible to enclose the whole wire antenna by a closed surface. As illustrated in Figure 2.19, the wire must pass through the "Huygens box" (i.e. the surface used in the implementation of the equivalent principle). In this case, as shown in [STR 41], and accordingly to section 2.2.6.1.2, additional charges have to be added. In this case, studies have shown that it is possible to cross the Huygens box. The results are stable, but the accuracy still needs to be improved [LAU 01].

We can conclude that the MoMTD-FDTD hybrid method is elegant but with a marginal use. This is due to the fact that, on the one hand, other methods (e.g. FDTD + MoM + SWE) can be used in case the antenna is far from the "diffractive object" and, on the other hand, because of the limited accuracy in the case antenna is linked to the "diffractive object".

2.3.4.4. *Homogenization*

2.3.4.4.1. Introduction

The FDTD grid mesh used in SAR assessment is often close to a millimeter because of the frequency bands used in wireless communication (e.g. 900, 1,800, 2,100, 2,400, 2,600 for 2G, 3G, 4G and WiFi systems) and anatomy but also, and often, mainly to take into account specific dielectric properties of tissues. Indeed, the dielectric permittivity and conductivity are influencing the electric field propagation in tissues but the spatial variations of the electric field are quite regular as shown. On the other hand, the conductivity is a major parameter for local SAR; for example, even if as shown in Figure 2.50 the E field strengths in gray brain matter and CSF are similar, the conductivities of these tissues are significantly different (respectively, 0.95 and 2.41 S/m) inducing significant different local SAR in CSF and the brain.

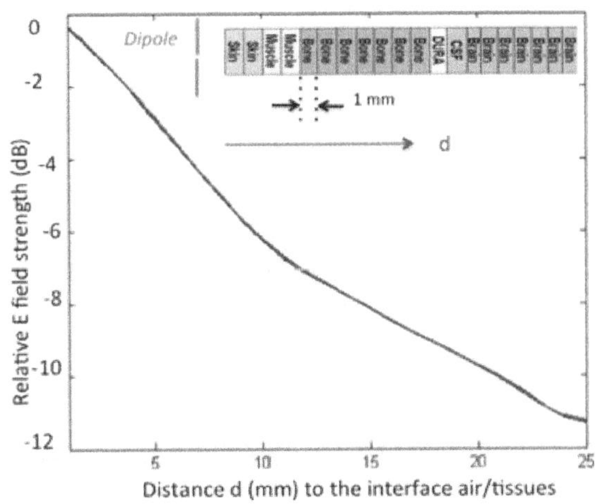

Figure 2.50. *Electric field in 1 mm layered head tissue model induced by a dipole operating at 900 MHz*

A tissue homogenization technique (THT) has been studied [EDC 08, EDC 08] to reduce the computational cost while keeping an acceptable accuracy of SAR assessment. THT can be an alternative to sub-gridding

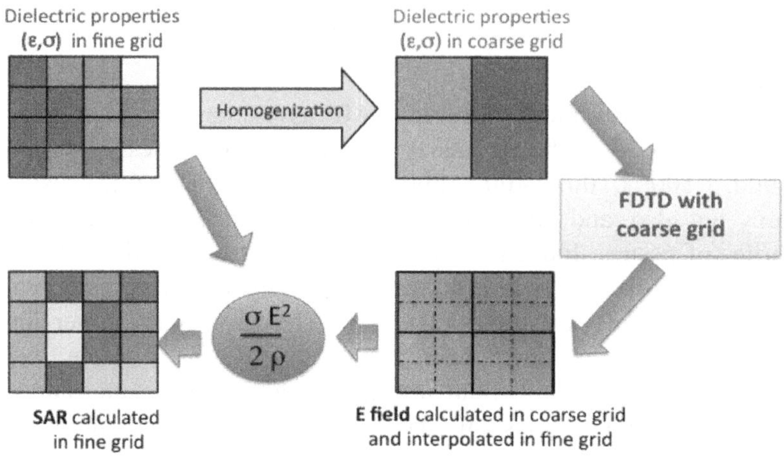

Figure 2.51. *Tissue homogenization technique applied to SAR assessment. For a color version of the figure, see www.iste.co.uk/wiart/radiofrequency.zip*

Figure 2.51 illustrates the THT principle. The biological object is defined in the fine mesh; the dielectric properties of the media in a coarse grid are derived from the dielectric properties of the media in the fine grid. These properties are used with FDTD to calculate the E field in the coarse grid. Their E field strength values are interpolated in the fine grid and used with the conductivity of media in the fine grid to estimate the SAR. The accuracy of the E field assessment and the impedance estimation using THT have been investigated and have shown quite good accuracy [LAU 00].

This THT method has been after that applied to assess the SAR induced by a frontal plane wave in the tissues of a child head [PRA 06] (head model developed within the ANR ADONIS project [BUR 04]). A “2 mm” resolution model has been derived from the 1 mm one. Figure 2.52 shows that fine details of the anatomy are modeled less in the coarse grid but global shapes are well preserved.

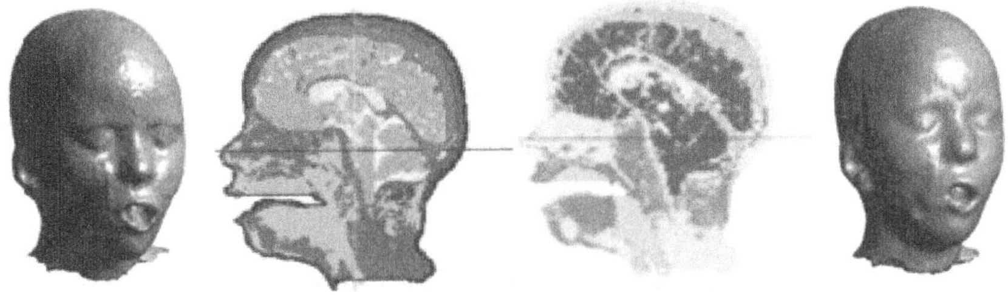

Figure 2.52. *Child head models with 1 mm (left) and 2 mm (right) resolution. For a color version of the figure, see www.iste.co.uk/wiart/radiofrequency.zip*

The 11 original tissue properties have been used to calculate, using averaging, the dielectric properties of 994 averaged tissues needed in the coarse grid having a 2 mm resolution. These values have come after those used in FDTD to assess the E field (see Figure 2.53).

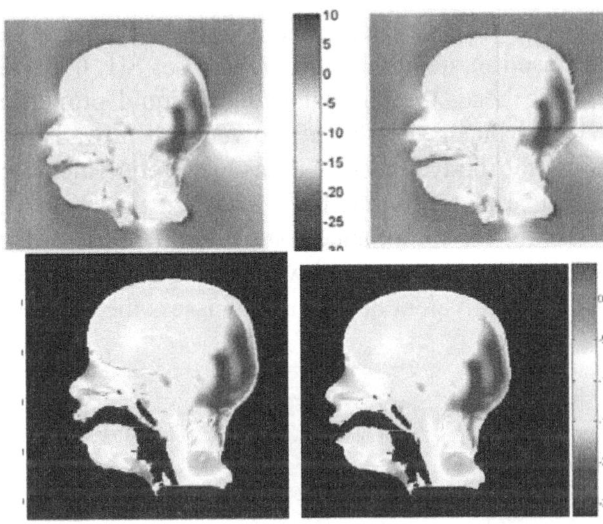

Figure 2.53. *E field, log scaling (upper line) and SAR, log scaling (lower line) calculated with 1 mm (left column) and 2 mm (right column) mesh resolution. For a color version of the figure, see www.iste.co.uk/wiart/radiofrequency.zip*

The differences have been analyzed (see Figure 2.54) and have shown that the relative error is less than 10% for 90% of the value.

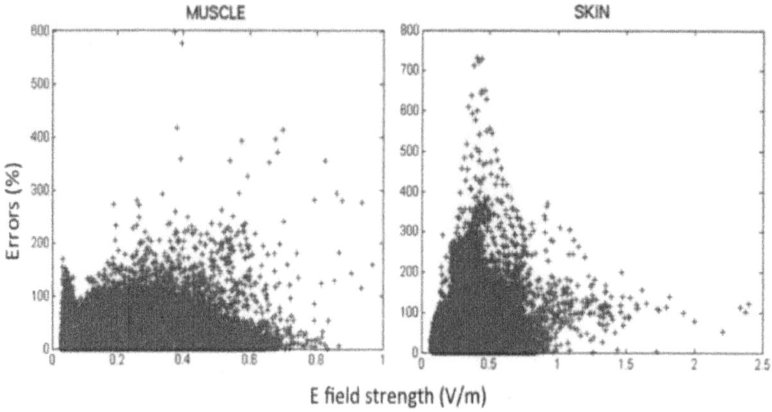

Figure 2.54. *Relative errors on electric field strength induced by a frontal plane wave operating at 900 MHz in head tissues model with 2 and 1 mm resolution*

Homogenization has also been used to specify the properties of the equivalent liquid used in standardization [PRA 06, SIL 09, PRA 08]. For a handset close to the head, the equivalent head liquid properties have been studied in the 1990s but usages have evolved and nowadays handsets are also used close to the body. In such a case, the equivalent liquid used to check the compliance to limits has been revisited to check if its dielectric properties are relevant for compliance test of mobile close to the bust, and if a correction factor (CF) has to be used when using the equivalent head liquid rather than a specific equivalent bust liquid to assess the 10 g averaged SAR.

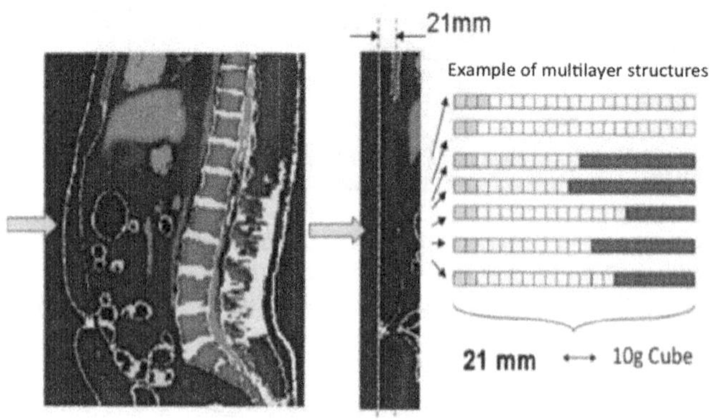

Figure 2.55. *Example of multilayers structure derived from visible human. For a color version of the figure, see www.iste.co.uk/wiart/radiofrequency.zip*

The bust tissues of the visible human have been analyzed and a total number of 176,749 multilayer structures have been derived (see Figure 2.55 for one structure). From these structures and their occurrence, 45 different combinations of tissues have been established and the tenth most encountered structures that are representing 54% of the total ones have been selected. These structures have been exposed to a field emitted by dipole located at various frequencies (0.9, 1.8, 2.1, 2.4 and 5.8 GHz) and distances (15 distances between 5 and 160 mm). To reduce the uncertainty linked to the dipole modeling, the electric field and the dipole impedance in tissues have been calculated using a method[7] based on MoMs through the determination of Green's function [DUD 95, MOS 84, WAI 96]. The SAR over 10 g in these structures has been compared to the SAR over 10 g obtained in the equivalent head liquid (see Figure 2.56). These results have been used to estimate the correction factor (CFi) that is the ratio between the 10 g averaged SAR calculated in the heterogeneous multilayer structure #i and the 10 g averaged SAR calculated in homogeneous equivalent head liquid. The CFi depends on the frequency and on the distance between the body and the sources. Figure 2.56 shows variations of CFi's with the distance. This figure also shows the limitation of too regular multilayers based on planes structures. Such model can induce phase and counter-phase interferences that cannot exist with biological tissues.

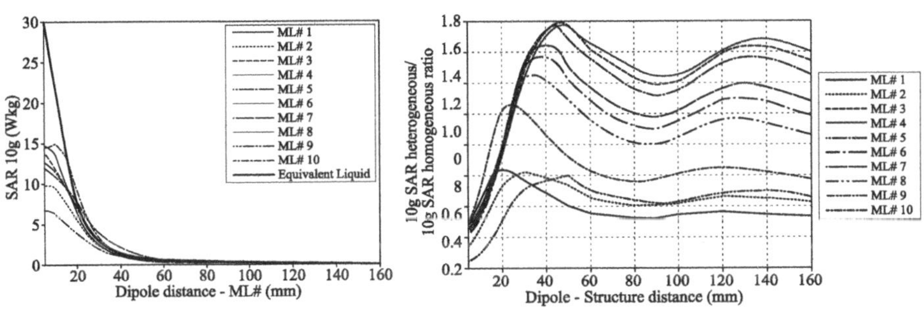

Figure 2.56. *Ten grams averaged SAR, normalized to 1 W input, induced by a dipole operating at 1,800 MHz in different structures (left) and CF for different ML at 1,800 MHz (right) versus distance from the dipole to the multilayers structures*

7 EM Software & Systems-Technopark, Stellenbosch 7600, PO Box 1354, Stellenbosch 7599, South Africa. Online: http://www.feko.info/.

As shown in Figure 2.56, the 10 g averaged SAR is a combination of 441 multilayer structures (the multilayer structures used in a cube of 21 × 21 × 21 mm^3. Taking into account the local occurrence of 441 multilayer structures involved in the 10 g averaged SAR, a local ratio LCF can be defined using the sum of the CFi's weighted using their occurrences.

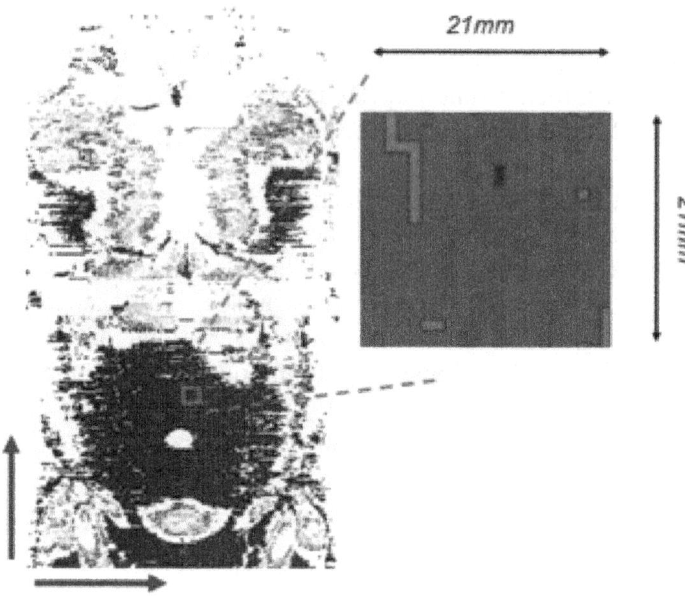

Figure 2.57. *Example of multilayer structures involved in a 10 g cube. For a color version of the figure, see www.iste.co.uk/wiart/radiofrequency.zip*

For each frequency and each distance, there is a maximum of the LCFi [SIL 08]. For all the frequencies, a global local ratio (GLR), defined as maximum of the maximum lCFi, can be estimated. This GLR provides a conservative ratio between SAR assessed in multilayers structures representing the human body and the SAR assessed in heterogeneous liquid. As shown in [SIL 09], this GLR is all the time less than 1.2. This study with other studies conducted at the international level has been used as a standard to validate the use of the equivalent head to assess the SAR in burst.

2.4. RF exposure assessment

2.4.1. *RF exposure to far source*

2.4.1.1. *Far source modeling*

When the sources are far from the location where the exposure has to be assessed, for instance a radio base station located on a building roof and a user located in the street, the source of exposure can be approximated by a plane wave or a sum of plane wave. In this case, the exposure assessment can be carried out using a plane wave and Huygens box [CHR 10, WU 11], based on the equivalent principle, as described in section 2.2.5.

2.4.1.2. *Exposure assessment*

As described in section 1.2.2.2, the relationship between the whole-body SAR and the incident field is a key question since the E field measurement is easier than the SAR one and thus such a relationship is used in standards. Because of this, a large effort has been made to characterize such a transfer function.

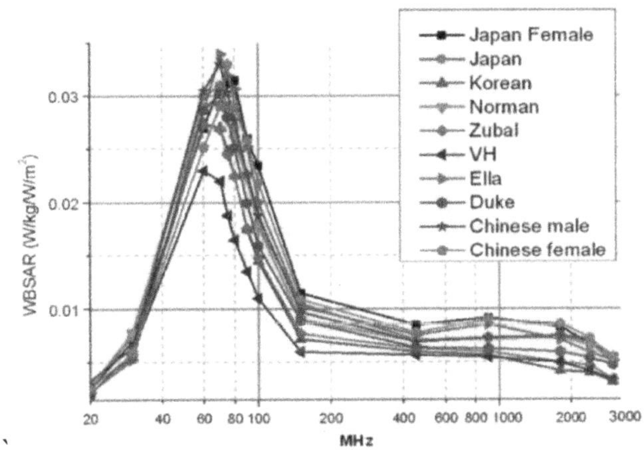

Figure 2.58. *Whole-body SAR versus frequency for different numerical human body models (after [WU 11]). For a color version of the figure, see www.iste.co.uk/wiart/radiofrequency.zip*

The whole-body SAR strongly depends on frequency bands (see Figure 2.58). Close to 100 MHz, where the human body size (between 1.5 and 2 m height) is close to a dipole having its resonance in this frequency band, a good efficiency for acquiring the energy can be observed. Close to 2 GHz, the influence of the frequency is much less important, and the whole-body SAR is linked to the human cross-section that varies between the individuals.

2.4.1.3. *Influence of morphology*

In the frequency bands between 60 and 100 MHz, where the human body size has a good efficiency (section 2.4.1.1) for obtaining the energy, the morphology also influences the whole-body exposure (see Figure 2.59). As Figure 2.59 shows, the morphology can have an important influence on the whole-body SAR induced by a frontal incident plane wave (± 40%).

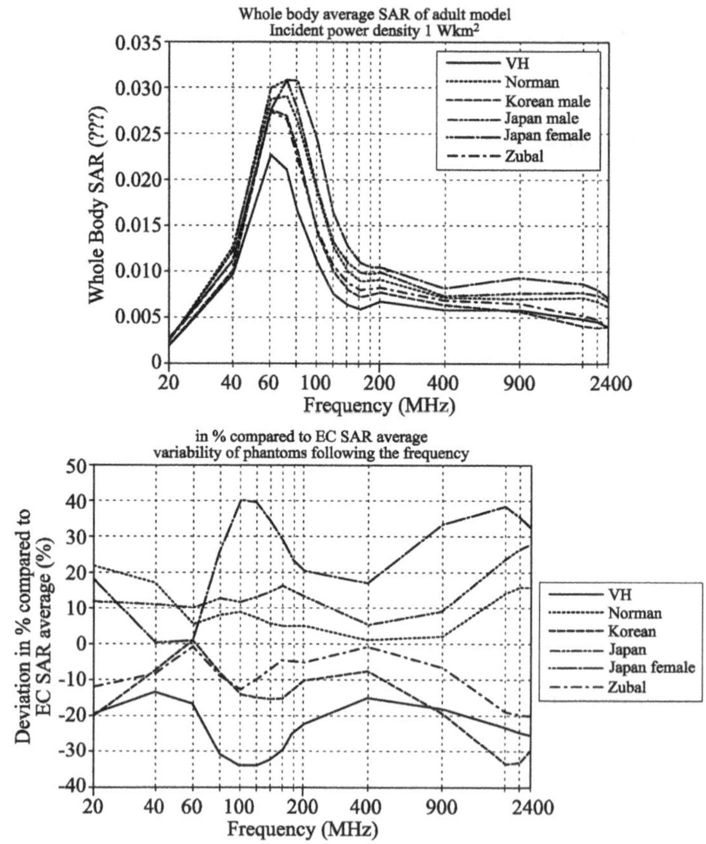

Figure 2.59. *Variability analysis of SAR from 20 MHz to 2.4 GHz*

To investigate the influence of children morphology on RF exposure, 5-, 8- and 12-year-old models built using piecewise scaling have been used [CON 11]. The compliance with a basic restriction of model exposed to reference levels has been studied. As shown in Figure 2.60, the whole-body SAR induced in small people can be higher than the one induced in large people.

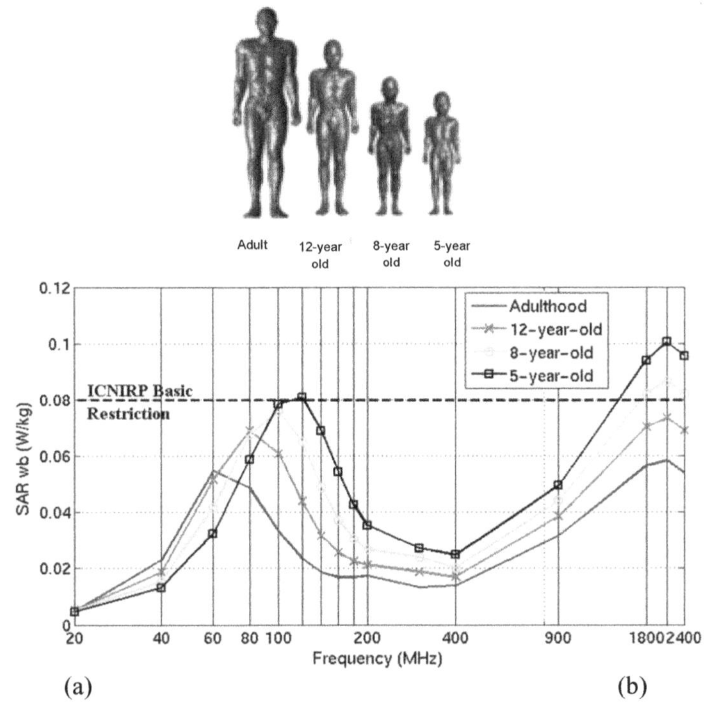

Figure 2.60. *Child models built with piecewise deformation a). Whole-body SAR of children model exposed to ICNIRP reference levels b). For a color version of the figure, see www.iste.co.uk/wiart/radiofrequency.zip*

2.4.1.4. *Influence of polarization and angle of arrival*

The influence of polarization and angle of influence can be determined with the Huygens box method. Figure 2.61 shows for the horizontal and vertical polarizations, at the frequency of 2.1 GHz, the influence of azimuth and elevation on plane wave exposure [CON 11]. The different behaviors for the V and H polarizations at 180° (i.e. plane wave coming from the back) can be explained by the flattening of the visible human model back, due to the position of the person during the acquisition of the images used to build the model.

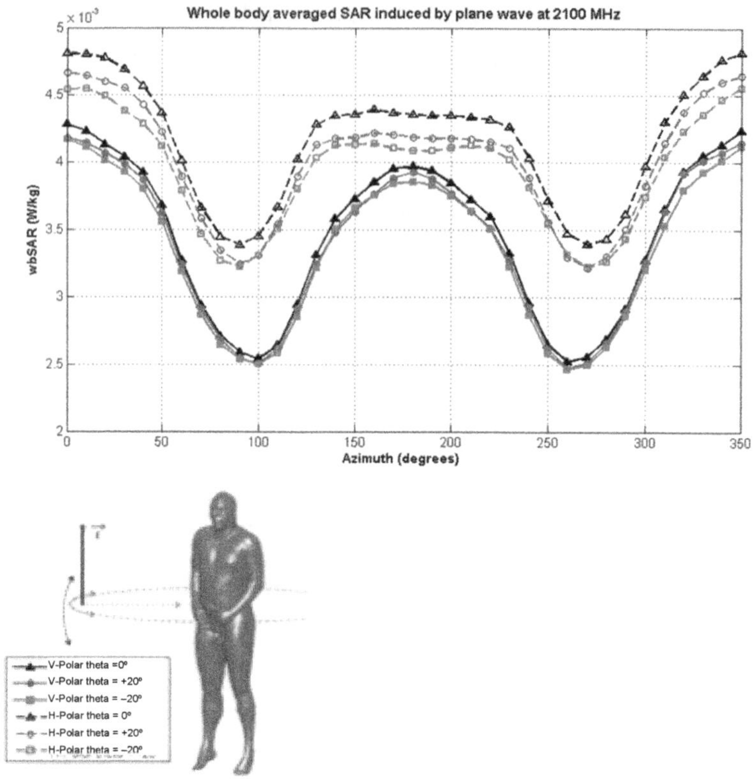

Figure 2.61. *Influence of the polarization, azimuth and elevation on whole-body SAR at 2.1 GHz. For a color version of the figure, see www.iste.co.uk/wiart/radiofrequency.zip*

2.4.2. *Exposure induced by a source in the near field*

2.4.2.1. *Source modeling*

WiFi boxes, small-cells and femtocells[8] are being increasingly used in network architectures. From the exposure point of view, the specificity of such systems is the proximity of humans with antennas that can be located at distances of 1 or 2 m from them. To perform the exposure assessment, an

8 http://en.wikipedia.org/wiki/Femtocell.

initial approach can be, basically, to model the source and use this source model with the human model in the FDTD computational domain. In this case, the FDTD domain would be big and the associated computational cost would be very long. If on the other hand we consider that the distance from the source to the human body is large enough to neglect the coupling, then the equivalent principle can be used but conversely to section 2.4.1 the source is in this case too close to consider *a priori* that the field emitted can be approximated by an incident plane wave. As described in section 2.2.6.3.2, the source can be modeled using spherical wave expansion (SWE) and used with a Huygens box.

2.4.2.2. *Example of exposure assessment to a femtocell*

To assess the exposure induced by a "Femto", the field emitted by this communication system can be measured and the coefficient of the SWE can be extracted (see section 2.2.6.3.2). Using this incident field described by SWE and the equivalence principle (see section 2.2.6.3), FDTD simulations can be performed to calculate the SAR.

This approach has been used to assess the exposure induced by a commercial 3G femto box emitting at 2,100 MHz. Measurements have been conducted to extract the coefficients Q_{smn} that characterize the emission of a femtocell system. Figure 2.62(c) shows the 3D radiation pattern of this femtocell, while Figures 2.62(a) and (b) shows that the radiation pattern is quite omnidirectional except for specific angles ($\theta = -180°$ and $\theta = -130°$; $\varphi = 190°$) corresponding to the bottom of the Femto antenna.

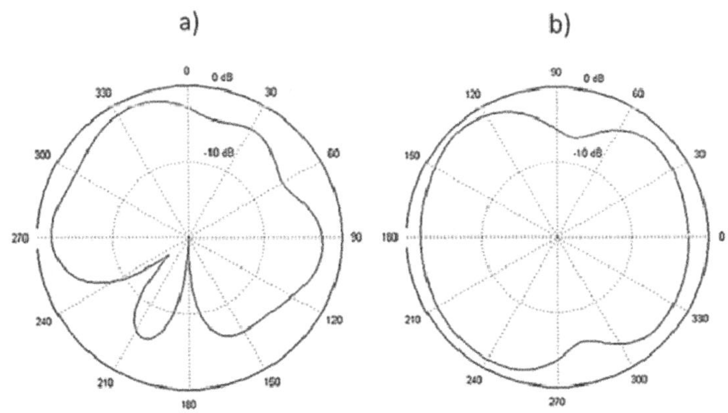

Figure 2.62. *Radiation patterns of the femtocell antenna versus* $\{\theta, \varphi\}$ *with* $\varphi = 0°$ *a) and* $\theta = 90°$ *b)*

Using the knowledge of the incident EMF emitted by the femto antenna in free space (via the SWE) and a Huygens box (see Figure 2.63), the SAR calculations can be performed, using FDTD, with different angles and distances. In the present case, the "frontal" exposure is defined by the angles $\theta = 90°$ and $\varphi = 0°$. Using the "Louis" body model, the whole-body SAR and the maximum 10 g averaged SAR induced by the femtocell and those induced by plane wave can be obtained. The exposure has been assessed with arbitrary input power: an input power of 1 W for the femtocell and a power density of 2.5 mW/m^2 for the plane wave.

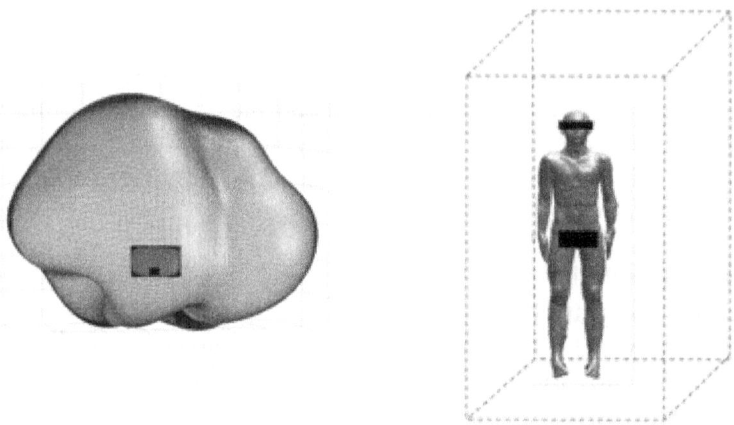

Figure 2.63. *Huygens box and Louis exposure (side exposure) to the femtocell*

Since power is a key parameter for the exposure, fair assessment or comparisons of the exposure require us to discuss the incident power density linked to the plane wave and the power radiated by the "Femto".

Considering the structure of the EMF as those of a plane wave has a lot of advantages since a large number of studies have been performed with the plane waves (e.g. [CHR 10, WU 11, ZUB 94]). It is therefore of interest to discuss the accuracy of such a simplification in case of a femtocell. The power radiated by the femtocell has been kept to 1 W while the E-field amplitude of the plane wave was set up to the rms E-field amplitude over the front face of the Huygens box. We can see with the comparisons shown by Figure 2.64 that the whole-body SAR relative error as well as the maximum 10 g averaged SAR relative error between the femtocell exposure and its plane wave approximation decreased with the increasing distance. The plane wave can be considered as an approximation continued overestimating the whole-body SAR.

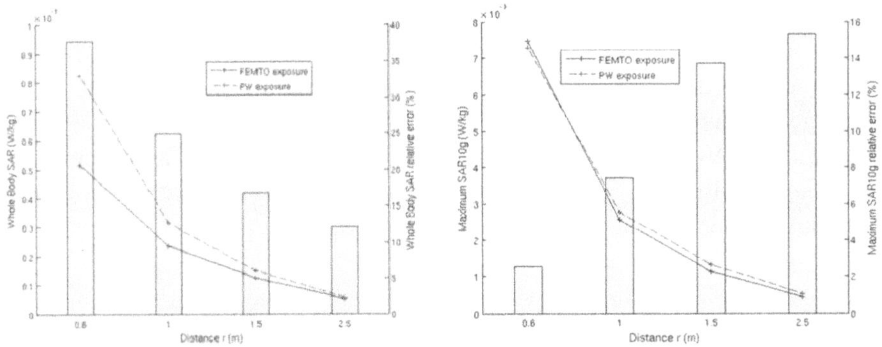

Figure 2.64. *Comparison of "Louis" whole-body SAR (left) and maximum 10 g averaged SAR (right) induced by a femtocell and plane wave at various distances. The absolute values are represented using lines with a left y-axis; the relative errors are represented using bars with a right y-axis*

For the maximum of the 10 g SAR, the plane wave approximation seems to be, for all distances, a good version of the maximum local exposure induced in the Louis model by the femtocell device. Nevertheless, the spatial distribution of the SAR induced by a femto in the body is not exactly the same as those induced by a plane wave. As shown in Figure 2.65, the location of the maximum 10 g averaged SAR is not the same even if at 2.5 m they are relatively close.

2.4.3. *Exposure induced by a source with tissues in the reactive field*

2.4.3.1. *Source modeling*

When the mobile is close to the head, unlike in sections 2.4.1 and 2.4.2, the biological tissues are in the reactive field. In such cases, there are possible interactions between the RF source and the tissues. Because of this, the equivalent principle cannot be used to calculate the exposure accurately and the source has to be modeled as the biological tissues. The complexity of an RF source close to the body can be highly variable. It can be a dipole antenna linked to a transmitter via a coaxial cable, it can be also a compact wireless system composed, as with a mobile phone, of a transmitter, an amplifier and an antenna. The first case is quite simple to model while the second one can be complex as pointed out in IEC 62704-3 [IEE 15a]. Indeed, a wireless communication system can be composed of different solids such as components, wires, screens, PCBs, batteries, and chassis that are not necessarily square boxes or easy to model with an orthogonal grid mesh (see Figure 2.66). To limit the computational effort, not all the components have to be modeled, for instance those that are inside shield-cans can be obviously removed. Conversely, others, such as antennas but also components such as displays, PCBs and batteries that have metallic parts, have to be modeled as accurately as possible.

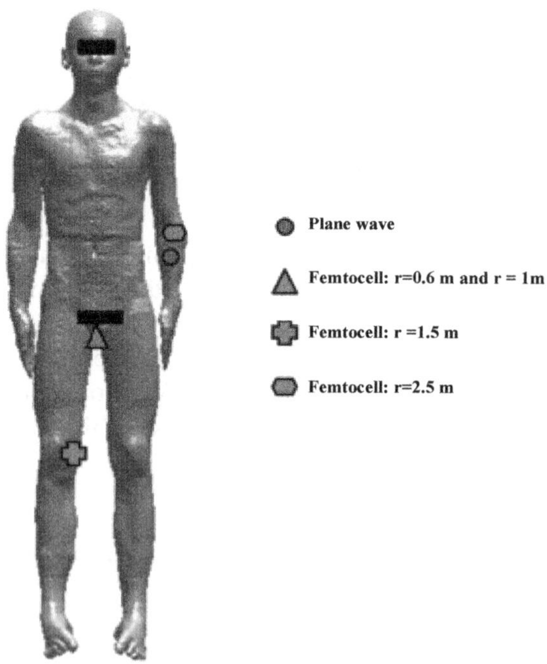

Figure 2.65. *Localization of the maximum 10 g SAR on the Louis model for femtocell and plane wave exposures*

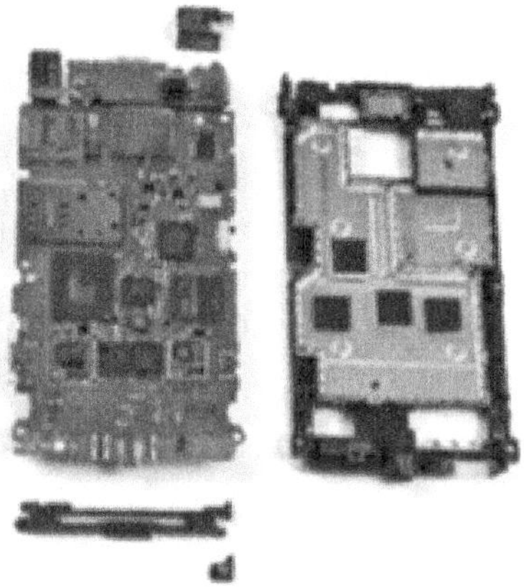

Figure 2.66. *View of internal circuits of a mobile phone*

The level of refinement in the model obviously depends on the objective. For instance, the design of a new commercial phone will require high levels of detail. In this case and because of the complexity of smartphones, the FDTD mesh is often generated by importation of the CAD file of the phone. In the case of epidemiological studies, the objective is not to design a phone and optimize a specific feature. The objective of the dosimetry in epidemiological studies is to assess the exposure induced by similar phones since accurately modeling all the existing phones is unrealistic; in this way, generic phones, representative classes of phone (e.g. bar phone, slide phone, antenna on the top, on the bottom, etc.), can be used [PIN 11]. Figure 2.67 shows an example of a simplified phone model.

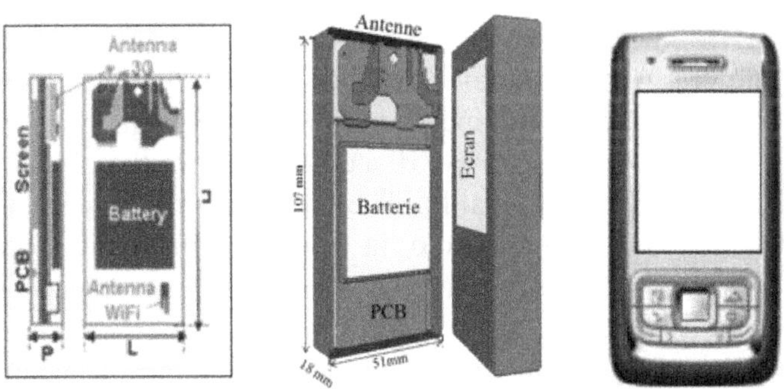

Figure 2.67. *Example of a simplified phone model of a similar commercial one. For a color version of the figure, see www.iste.co.uk/wiart/radiofrequency.zip*

In any case, the model of the handset has to be verified; on the one hand, the critical areas such as the antenna shape, gap (where the input RF energy is provided) and other conductive components, on the other hand, the behavior of the antenna. The return loss S11 that quantifies how much power is reflected from the antenna has to be calculated through the impedance: if S11 is too close to zero, nothing is radiated. Figure 2.68 shows that the S11 of the phone model shown in Figure 2.67 is acceptable in the frequency band of interest.

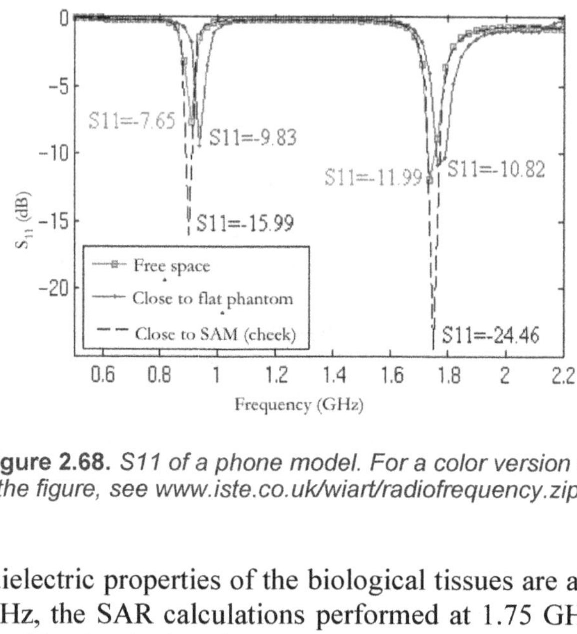

Figure 2.68. *S11 of a phone model. For a color version of the figure, see www.iste.co.uk/wiart/radiofrequency.zip*

Since the dielectric properties of the biological tissues are about the same over ± 100 MHz, the SAR calculations performed at 1.75 GHz are valid at 1.8 or 1.9, the objective is therefore not, conversely to a commercial phone design, to have a phone model operating at an exact frequency but to run the FDTD calculation at the frequency, if acceptable from the objective point of view, where the S11 is acceptable. The SAR distribution is also of great interest and must be also checked in SAM or in a flat phantom. The normalized SAR (to the maximum), induced by the simplified phone (SAR assessed using FDTD calculations) and a similar phone (SAR assessed using measurements) located 5 mm from the liquid filling the flat phantom are, as shown in Figure 2.69, very similar. Some metrics have been studied [GHA 13] to compare the discrepancies.

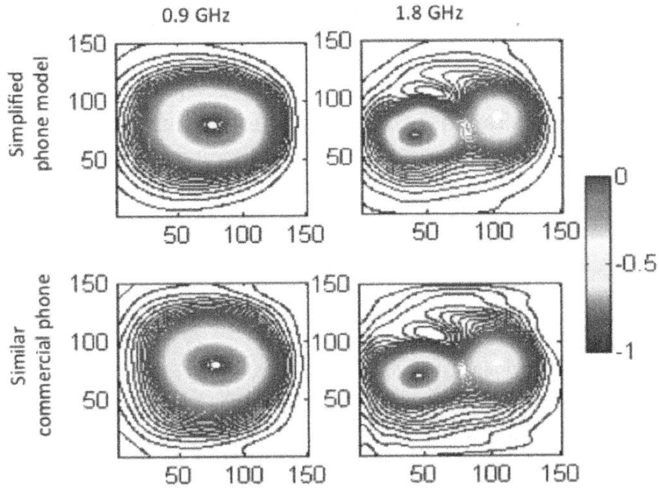

Figure 2.69. *Comparison between SAR, normalized to the maximum, induced by a simplified numerical phone model (via FDTD) and induced by a similar commercial one (via measurement). For a color version of the figure, see www.iste.co.uk/wiart/radiofrequency.zip*

2.4.3.2. *Influence of a handset phone position on RF exposure of brain tissues*

As mentioned out in Chapter 1, the 1990s and 2000s have seen an unprecedented increase in the use of wireless communicating devices. To protect the general public from overexposure, standards have been adopted to guarantee the compliance of product put on the market. Despite this process, the questions have continued to exist and have asked biomedical and epidemiological studies about their conclusions regarding possible risk (on EMF). The epidemiological studies have a specific status since they directly address the exposure and disease occurrence in the population. The international epidemiological studies that have been carried out (e.g. projects "Cephalo", "Interphone", "Cosmos", "Mobi-kids" and "Geronimo" [AHL 05, CAR 10, SCH 11]) have focused on brain exposure because of the questions linked to the proximity, during the voice calls, of the phone to these tissues. As a consequence, brain exposure assessment has been a key question for these studies and investigated in several studies [KAI 05, BEA 08, KUS 04] with the phone in cheek or tilt position. Brain tissue exposure has been investigated using a measurement performed in SAM homogeneous liquid or using numerical phone model and heterogeneous head models [GOS 11, GHA 14]. As we can expect, the exposure of brain areas depends on the location of the antenna.

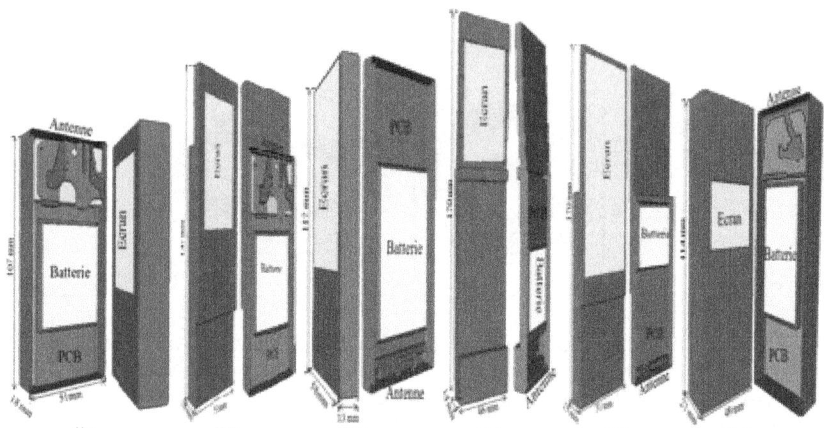

Figure 2.70. *Different phone models having antenna on the top (#1, #6), in the middle (#2) and at the bottom (#3, #4, #5) For a color version of the figure, see: www.iste.co.uk/wiart/radiofrequency.zip*

To characterize such influence, studies have been carried out [GOS 11, GHA 13] using the "Duke" adult heterogeneous head model (described in section 2.3.2.2) and using several phone models [PIN 13], shown in Figure 2.70, designed in the ANR project Kidpocket (http://whist.institut-telecom.fr). These phones are representative of devices having different antenna locations (on the top, in the middle or at the bottom). The exposure induced in the head by these different phone models has been calculated using FDTD. Figure 2.71 shows the E field radiated by the different phones.

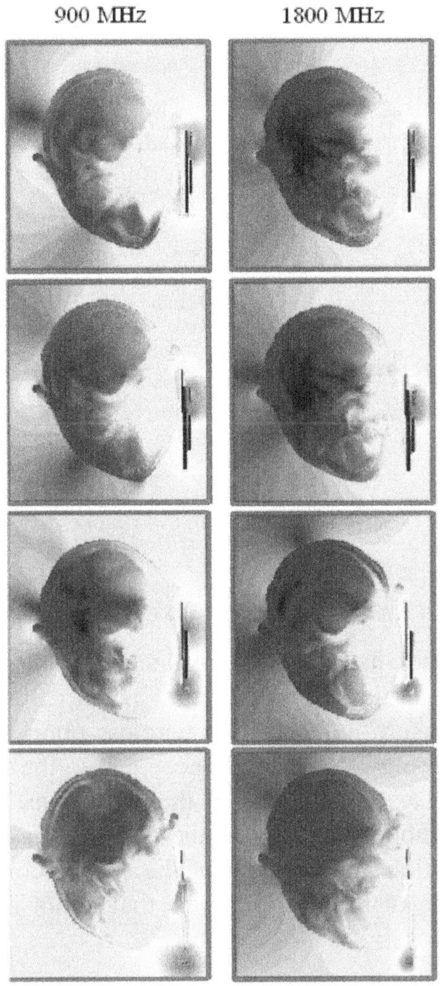

Figure 2.71. *Exposure induced by the different phone models at different frequencies. For a color version of the figure, see www.iste.co.uk/wiart/radiofrequency.zip*

Figure 2.72 shows the average SAR in different anatomical brain structures with an input power (Pin) such that the SAR 10 g reaches 1 W/kg within the SAM phantom [IEC 05] in the cheek position. In a "voice" posture (i.e. the mobile phone close to the ear), the main exposed area is the temporal lobe as we can expect.

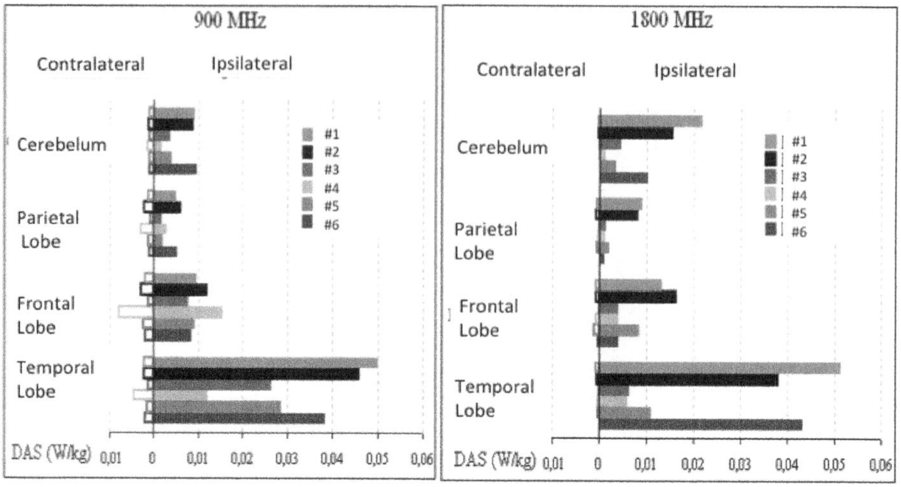

Figure 2.72. *Duke brain tissue exposure with the mobile phone in the cheek position*

2.4.3.3. *Influence of the phone position on the emitted power*

The previous section has shown the influence of the position of the phone and its antenna on brain exposure. But, as explained in sections 1.2.4 and 1.2.4.1, the exposure induced by a wireless phone also depends on the power emitted. During the compliance tests, the power emitted by the equipment being tested is set up at the maximum. But the usual power emitted by cellular phones depends on the network and on the environment, the base station location and the gain of the couple composed of the user's body and the antenna of the user's device that is not isotropic as shown in Figure 2.73.

To keep the signal-to-noise ratio close to the target value (see section 1.2.4.1), the power emitted by the phone varies inversely to the variations of the gain. At a given distance, the previous constraint means that the product of the power supplied to the antenna (Pe) and the transmitting antenna gain (Ge) should be constant. In case of free space, as shown in Figure 2.73, there is only one path and the power emitted is as (equation [2.92]):

$$P_e(\theta_{LOS}, \varphi_{LOS}) = \frac{Cst}{G_e(\theta_{LOS}, \varphi_{LOS})} \qquad [2.92]$$

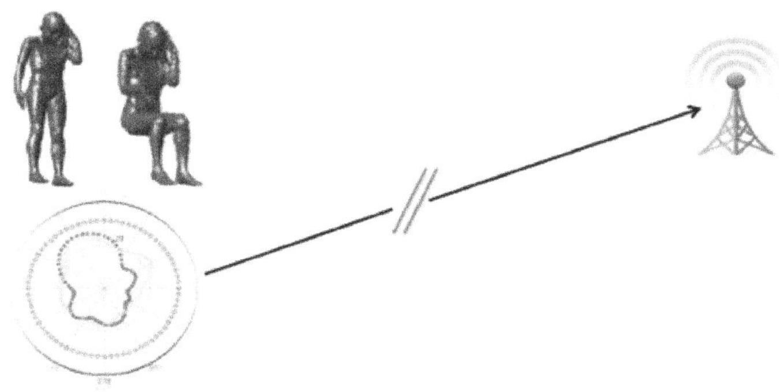

Figure 2.73. *Gain of the couple composed of the user's body (in standing and sitting positions) and the antenna of the user's device*

The antenna performance has been studied [KRA 16] by the characterization of the power emitted by the antennas under specific propagation assumptions. A realistic numerical model of child body, the Eartha child body model [CHR 10], has been used in three different postures usages of wireless devices operating at 900 and 1,940 MHz. The effects of the human body on the variability of the effective gain are carried out using an FDTD method.

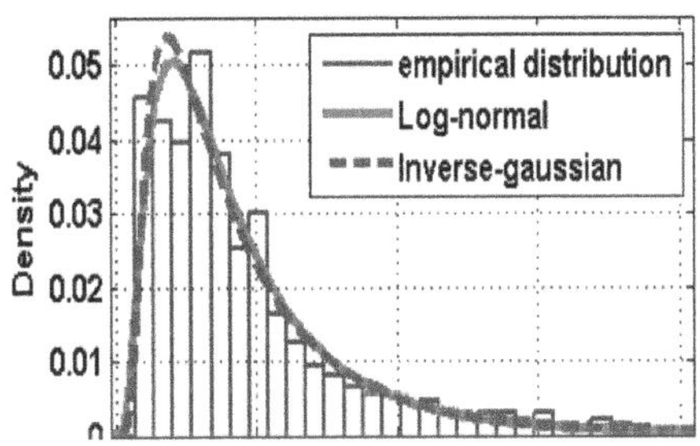

Figure 2.74. *Distribution density of the propagation gain of the couple composed of the user's body (in standing and sitting positions) and the antenna of the user's device. For a color version of the figure, see www.iste.co.uk/wiart/radiofrequency.zip*

2.5. Conclusion

The numerical methods applied to electromagnetism have taken advantage of the progress in HPC. This chapter describes the main features of the FDTD, the dispersion, the stability, the absorbing boundary condition such as the PML and the calculation of the SAR. This chapter shows how to model the sources using 3D spatial modeling, thin structures and equivalent principles using a Huygens box with a plane wave and spherical mode. This chapter provides dosimetric calculations for adult and child RF exposure.

Because of the versatile use of wireless communication systems, numerical dosimetry is facing a new challenge: complexity and the variability. The posture, morphology and source location cannot be considered as constant as they are varying. The SAR is therefore not a value but a statistical distribution. Even if the numerical dosimetry has been improved today, computer capabilities do not allow computing thousands of simulations since the duration of one simulation is still significant. Because of this, a new domain has been opened: namely, stochastic dosimetry. The third chapter will introduce this domain.

3

Stochastic Dosimetry

"As far as the laws of mathematics refer to reality, they are not certain; and as far as they are certain, they do not refer to reality".

Albert EINSTEIN

3.1. Motivations

The two previous chapters have presented, on the one hand, human RF exposure and the wireless communication system and, on the other hand, computational electromagnetics applied to human exposure assessment. With the versatile use of wireless communication systems and with the increasing use of wireless connected objects (e.g. smart meters, sensors) with different communication protocols (GSM, UMTS, LTE and WiFi but also new approaches such as Low Power Wide Area (LPWA), the deterministic approaches are facing strong limitations due to varying postures, anatomy, technologies, etc.

This chapter is dedicated to stochastic methods applied to human exposure assessment and the recent trends in numerical methods to use statistics to assess RF exposure.

To cope with the increasing and versatile use of wireless devices, much research has been carried out to create realistic human phantoms (see section 2.3.2) with millimeter resolutions. Adult, child and fetus medical images have been analyzed and segmented to create voxel models. To handle the versatile uses of RF devices and their users's postures, efforts have also been performed to build deformation tools applicable to numerical human models. Despite these significant efforts over recent decades, the challenge still exits. For instance, several phantom models have been designed, but even in the same age classification (e.g. adults), the morphology is highly variable (section 2.3.2.4) and brings a large variability of exposure (section 2.4.1.3). The RF source location and the user postures reinforce this trend.

Characterizing such variable exposure with the usual dosimetric numerical methods (e.g. finite difference in time domain (FDTD)) can require a very large number of simulations. In spite of the progress observed during the past decade in high-performance calculation, the simulations still require computation times that are not compatible with Monte Carlo (MC) simulation. To respond to this challenge, a new domain has appeared in recent years in RF exposure assessment: stochastic dosimetry [WIA 04].

The main idea of stochastic dosimetry is to use statistic tools to build a surrogate model able to replace the heavy numerical solver by analytical equations that are as simple as possible that are able to provide results very quickly. This surrogate model can be used to obtain, parsimoniously, the distribution of the quantity of interest (whole body or organ specific absorption rate (SAR) for instance); it can also be used to perform a sensitivity analysis (SA) and characterize the statistical variations of the output brought about by the variation in the inputs.

3.2. The challenge of variability for numerical dosimetry

As discussed in earlier sections, numerical RF exposure assessment is at present facing new challenges in coping with the variability of usages and assessing the uncertainty of numerical calculations obtained in specific configurations. SAR caused by a phone in brain tissue has been investigated by several studies [WIA 11, WIA 08, DIM 94, GOS 11]. These have shown that tissue exposure depends not only on input parameters such as human morphology and anatomy [CON 08, ELH 10, WIA 08] but also on the dielectric properties of these tissues [GAB 10] that can be affected by a wide variability since they are highly non-homogeneous, possibly affected by age [GOS 11] and, for tissues such as skin, by external conditions. In addition to these parameters, the exposure also depends on phone design, antenna location, frequency and power emitted linked to the technologies [WIA 00, GAT 09].

To comply with a conservative approach, worst case scenarios have often been used to manage such variability, in particular in standardization programs. However, public information or epidemiological studies are not satisfied by such worst cases and request the assessment of the variation in "real" exposure. This needs to handle the influence on the exposure of the variable inputs.

In the absence of closed-form solutions to describe a physical phenomenon such as RF exposure, the MC method is often used in engineering problems to characterize the distribution of an unknown probabilistic entity. This MC method is also often used to estimate the numerical integration of complex functions. The MC uses random draws of a process to obtain the value of the function (that can be the distribution of an unknown probabilistic entity).

Consider a quantity y linked to the input x by equation [3.1], where y is the whole body SAR, x is the dielectric properties of tissues of a phantom and M is the physical model (e.g. the FDTD)

$$y = \mathcal{M}(x) \qquad [3.1]$$

Let us note the mean value m_y and the standard deviation S_y and assuming a sample of n input vectors $\{x(1), x(2), \ldots x(n)\}$, the usual estimators of the mean and standard deviation are given by [3.2] and [3.3]

$$m_y = \frac{1}{n} \sum_{i=1}^{n} \mathcal{M}(x^{(i)}) \qquad [3.2]$$

$$s_y = \sqrt{\frac{1}{(n-1)} \sum_{i=1}^{n} (\mathcal{M}(x^{(i)}) - m_y)^2} \qquad [3.3]$$

Because of the central limit theorem, the estimator, m_y, is asymptotically Gaussian. As a result, if n is sufficiently large, with $q_{1-\alpha/2}$ the α quantile of the centered and reduced Gaussian law $\mathcal{N}(0,1)$, the uncertainty of the estimator is given by $\pm q_{1-\alpha/2}\frac{S_y}{\sqrt{n}}$.

For example with a typical risk value of α = 5% the confidence interval of the mean is given by $m_y - 1.96\frac{S_y}{\sqrt{n}} \leq m \leq m_y + 1.96\frac{S_y}{\sqrt{n}}$. Similar formulas exist for the confidence interval of the standard deviation.

The main advantage of the MC method is its simplicity and its applicability to a large class of problems required but its main limitation is the very large number of experiments, for problems involving a large number of inputs or for higher mode estimation. Other methods exist [SUD 07] but they are also based on a large number of samples that are not compatible with numerical methods requiring large computation time such as the FDTD.

The main advantage of the FDTD is the ability to proceed without any matrix inversion, but the main constraint is the computation time, which can be very significant (i.e. a few hours if calculation involved the whole body) for human RF exposure assessment.

Much effort has been made toward high-performance computing using parallel architectures with recent graphic processor units. But even with these efforts, the computation time is still significant and is not compatible with the MC method, which requires a few hundred to a few thousand simulations depending on the required precision of the higher computed moments of the probability distribution.

3.3. Stochastic dosimetry and polynomial chaos expansion

3.3.1. *Surrogate models and numerical dosimetry*

The problem described in the earlier section is not specific to RF electromagnetic exposure assessment; it also occurs in engineering problems involving computer simulations requiring significant computation time.

Typical examples can be found in mechanics with the design optimization of an optimal shape. Indeed, for many real-world problems, a single simulation, as in RF dosimetry or in antenna design, can take several minutes or hours. Similar problems occur when the objective is to characterize the influence of inputs variations on the statistical distribution of the calculated outputs through the simulations.

One way to overcome such a limitation is to build simpler approximation models, known as alternative models, surrogate models, response surfaces or meta-models, which mimic the complex response of the model (represented in dosimetry by the FDTD simulations) as close as possible, while being inexpensive to calculate[1].

A model of a physical problem or system can be represented using a general function $\mathcal{M}: x \to y = \mathcal{M}(x)$ where x is a vector composed of the input parameters of the model ($x \in D \subset \mathbb{R}^{M}$). The model response, $y = \mathcal{M}(x)$, is also a vector with a dimension possibly different from the input. Within this formalism, described in Figure 3.1, the objective is to build an approximation of the model response: $\hat{y} = \widehat{\mathcal{M}}(x)$.

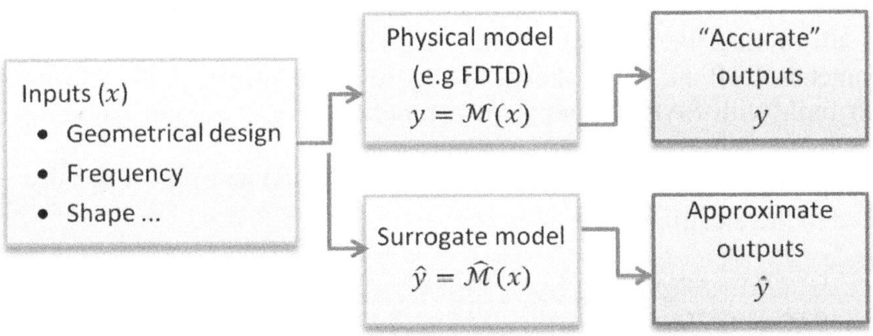

Figure 3.1. *General scheme for surrogate model use*

The construction of the surrogate model, $\widehat{\mathcal{M}}$, often considers the physical model (in our case, the FDTD simulator) as a "black box". Only the input–output relationship is considered to be important, the internal operations of the simulation code and the physical phenomena do not need to be known or

1 See http://www.openturns.org.

understood (i.e. the computer code pre-exists and must be used as it is). The main challenge is therefore to build the surrogate model $\widehat{\mathcal{M}}$ using the response of the simulator for a number of points that have to be selected so as to minimize this number relative to the objectives fixed for the surrogate model.

Once the surrogate model is built and validated, the issue of computation time is no longer a limit and the propagation of the uncertainties or the variability of the input data and the characterization of the outputs (shape of the distribution, quantiles and sensitivity) can be conducted using the MC method. Among the methods that exist to build these metamodels, we will look more specifically at regression, the Kriging method and polynomial chaos expansion (PCE) also known as "polynomial chaos" (PC). These methods have shown their great abilities to manage the kind of problems that dosimetry is facing. The construction of surrogate models imposes a sample of the real phenomenon that the simplified model tries to approximate. The following section discusses the method to select the experiments.

3.3.2. *Example of basic surrogate modeling in dosimetry*

Studies have been performed [CON 11] to simplify exposure assessment by substituting the visible human model into an ellipsoid. Using the parameters L, P and H as shown in Figure 3.2, a surrogate model [3.4] has been built with SAR as output of a function of the azimuth angle, ϕ; the morphological parameters, L, P and H; and the incident power density $\frac{E^2}{120\pi}$ linked to the electric field *E*.

$$\mathrm{SAR} = 0.75\frac{\pi\sqrt{\left(\frac{L}{2}\right)^2\cos(\phi)^2+\left(\frac{LP}{2}\right)^2\sin(\phi)^2}}{\frac{1}{3}LP\rho}\frac{E^2}{120\pi} \qquad [3.4]$$

This surrogate modeling is based on physical observation and took into account physical phenomena. In the present case, the concept of the equivalent surface of an antenna and the cross-section of the body has been used to build the surrogate model. Such knowledge is not always accessible and the phenomenon is not always as simple. For this reason, a general and generic approach is needed.

a)

b)

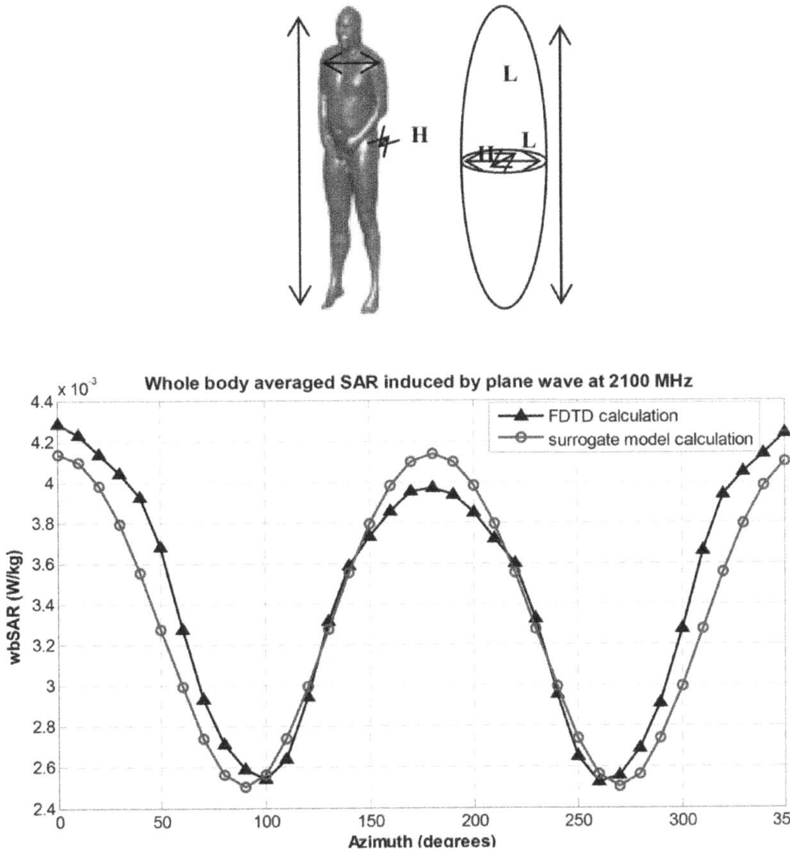

Figure 3.2. *a) L, P and H input parameters of the surrogate model; b) comparison between SAR calculation with FDTD and surrogate of the whole body SAR at 2.1 GHz*

3.4. PC and numerical dosimetry

In electromagnetics, the Kriging and the Gaussian process has been used in EMC problems [DEH 00] and in environmental *E* field exposure assessment [OUL 07, OUL 08, JAW 12, JAW 14]. Methods based on the stochastic finite element were introduced [CHA 06, XIU 05] in recent decades. These methods have already been used in other fields such as mechanics and fluid dynamics to incorporate random fluctuations in the deterministic finite-element method. The Kriging approach makes it possible to have a confidence interval of the surrogate model predictions. From the dosimetry point of view, the advantages of the stochastic finite elements and the PC, in particular, are, on the one hand, to be closer to the modal approaches used in electromagnetism and, on the other hand, to allow SA without additional calculations.

The key results on which the PC are based are due to Norbert Wiener [WIE 38] where Hermite polynomials were used to model stochastic processes with Gaussian random variables. Cameron and Martin [CAM 47] showed that such an expansion converges ($\mathcal{L}^2$) for any arbitrary stochastic process with a finite second moment.

Having a finite second moment is not a strong constraint in the engineering domain since most of the physical systems comply with it. Recent studies [GHA 91, SHO 00] have contributed to the development and use of stochastic methods in the engineering domain and have provided a mathematical framework to manage the variability of the inputs in numerical calculations.

The methods that use PC expansion can be divided into large categories. On the one hand, the intrusive methods requiring modification of the simulation code of the solver, and on the other hand, non-intrusive methods that use solvers as black boxes.

The first category, composed of the intrusive methods, requires manipulation of the governing equations and modification of the simulation software. This can be very complex and analytically cumbersome. The complexity of the intrusive approaches can explain the increasing attention given to the non-intrusive methods. These approaches use the complex codes as black boxes and can be easily generalizable.

The non-intrusive approaches are themselves composed of two categories: stochastic collocation and stochastic spectral methods. The stochastic collocation method constraints the polynomial approximation to exactly fit the physical response at a suitable point set. They rely upon well-established results on Lagrange polynomial interpolation [ABR 72]. With the stochastic spectral methods, the PC coefficients are estimated using spectral projections or least-square regressions.

In this section, we will pay specific attention to these spectral methods and their application to analyze the variations of the SAR (whole body or local) induced by the variations of the inputs.

Let us consider a mathematical model $\mathcal{M}$ having M inputs, $y = \mathcal{M}(x)$, with the inputs x affected by some possible random variations or uncertainties. Due to this, a probabilistic framework needs to be defined. Let us also note the probability space $(\Omega, \mathcal{F}, \mathcal{P})$, where Ω is the event space equipped with σ-algebra F and probability measure $\mathcal{P}$. In the following, M random variables are noted by upper case letters (ω): $\Omega \longrightarrow \mathcal{D}_X \subset \mathbb{R}^M$; their realizations are noted by the corresponding lower case letters (e.g. x).

Let us also note $\mathcal{L}^2(\Omega, \mathcal{F}, \mathcal{P}, \mathbb{R})$ the space of square-integrable real-valued functions equipped with the inner product [3.5]:

$$
\begin{aligned}
&< X_1, X_2 >_{\mathcal{L}^2_{\mathbb{R}}} \equiv E[X_1, X_2] \\
&= \int_{\Omega} X_1(\omega) X_2(\omega) d\mathcal{P}(\omega) \\
&= \int_{\mathcal{D}_X} x_1 x_2 f_{X_1,X_2}(x_1, x_2) dx_1 dx_2
\end{aligned}
\qquad [3.5]
$$

In [3.5], f_{X_1,X_2} is the joint probability density function (PDF) of the vector $\{X_1, X_2\}$. The inner product defines a norm ($\|X\| \equiv \sqrt{E(X^2)}$).

Let us consider a scalar-valued model M, e.g. the SAR calculated with the FDTD [3.7],

$$
\begin{aligned}
\mathcal{M}:\ & \mathbb{R}^M && \longmapsto \mathbb{R} \\
& X(\omega) && \longmapsto Y(\omega) = \mathcal{M}(X(\omega))
\end{aligned}
\qquad [3.6]
$$

with a finite second-order moment $E(Y^2) < +\infty$.

Then, $Y(\omega) = \mathcal{M}(X(\omega))$ can be described [SOI 04] using an infinite modal expansion [3.7]:

$$Y(\omega) = \sum_{\alpha \in \mathbb{N}^M} \beta_\alpha \psi_\alpha(X(\omega)) \qquad [3.7]$$

In [3.7], α are the multi-indices, ψ_α is the multidimensional orthogonal polynomials and β_α are the coefficients of the polynomial expansion. The presence of ω shows that the input X and the output Y are random variables. Formula [3.7] is the PCE of Y.

Assuming the independence of the input variables, the PDF of $X(\omega) = \{X_1(\omega), X_2(\omega), .. X_i(\omega), .. X_M(\omega)\}$ can be obtained using the marginal probability density [3.8]

$$f_X(x) = \prod_{i=1}^{M} f_{X_i}(x_i) \qquad [3.8]$$

In [3.8], $f_{X_i}(x_i)$ are the marginal PDF of X_i .

Let us now denote $\left\{\pi_j^{(i)}(X_i)\right\}$ the family of orthonormal polynomials with respect to $f_{X_i}(x_i)$, and having a degree j satisfying [3.9]

$$\langle \pi_j^{(i)}(X_i), \pi_k^{(i)}(X_i) \rangle = E\left(\pi_j^{(i)}(X_i), \pi_k^{(i)}(X_i)\right) = \delta_{j,k} \qquad [3.9]$$

where $\delta_{j,k}$ is the Kronecker symbol.

The tensorization of univariate polynomials provides a set of orthonormal multivariate polynomials $\{\psi_\alpha, \alpha \in \mathbb{N}^M\}$ where α denotes all the M-uplets $(\alpha_1, \alpha_2, \dots, \alpha_M) \in \mathbb{N}^M$ and ψ_α is defined by [3.10]

$$\psi_\alpha(x) = \prod_{i=1}^{M} \pi_{\alpha_i}^{(i)}(x_i) \qquad [3.10]$$

As explained previously, the PCE was originally formulated with standard Gaussian random variables and Hermite polynomials that are orthogonal with a Gaussian PDF (see equations [3.5] and [3.9]). This approach has been extended to other classical random variables together with basis functions. In this case, formula [3.7] is known as the generalized PCE of Y. Table 3.1 provides the associated family of polynomials for some of the most common continuous distributions.

Distribution	Density function	Support	Polynomial
Gaussian	$\frac{1}{\sqrt{2\pi}}e^{-x^2/2}$	$]-\infty,+\infty[$	*Hermite*: $H_{e_k}(x)$
Uniform	$1_{[-1,1]}(x)/2$	$[-1,+1]$	*Legendre*: $P_k(x)$
Gamma	$x^a e^{-x} 1_{\mathbb{R}+}(x)$	$[0,+\infty[$	*Laguerre*: $L_k^a(x)$
Beta	$1_{[-1,1]}(x)\frac{(1-x)^a(1+x)^b}{B(a)B(b)}$	$[-1,+1]$	*Jacobi*: $J_k^{a,b}(x)$

Table 3.1. *Example of relationship between families of orthogonal polynomials in generalized polynomial chaos expansion and usual input distributions*

The Gaussian and uniform distributions are often used in engineering; their associated polynomial families are the Hermite polynomial family $\{H_{e_k}(x)\}$ and the Legendre polynomial family $\{P_k(x)\}$. The Legendre family can be built using iterative formulas [3.11]–[3.14].

$$P_{-1}(x) \equiv P_0(x) = 1 \qquad [3.11]$$

$$(n+1)P_{n+1}(x) = (2n+1)xP_n(x) - nP_{n-1}(x) \;, n \in \mathbb{N} \qquad [3.12]$$

$$\int_{-\infty}^{+\infty} P_k(x)P_l(x)1_{[-1,1]}(x)1_{[-1,1]}(x)/2 = \frac{1}{2k+1}\delta_{k,l} \qquad [3.13]$$

$$P_0(x) = 1,\; P_1(x) = x,\; P_2(x) = \tfrac{1}{2}(3x^2-1)\,, P_3(x) = \tfrac{1}{2}(5x^3-3x), \qquad [3.14]$$

As for the Hermite family, the formulas are [3.16]–[3.18].

$$H_{e-1}(x) \equiv H_{eo}(x) = 1 \qquad [3.15]$$

$$H_{e_{n+1}}(x) = xH_{e_n}(x) - nH_{e_{n-1}}(x) \;, \quad n \in \mathbb{N} \qquad [3.16]$$

$$\int_{-\infty}^{+\infty} H_{e_k}(x) H_{e_l}(x) \frac{1}{\sqrt{2\pi}} e^{-x^2/2} dx = 1!\,\delta_{k,l} \qquad [3.17]$$

$$H_{e_0}(x) = 1,\ P_1(x) = x,\ H_{e_2}(x) = (x^2 - 1),\ H_{e_3}(x) = (x^3 - 3x) \qquad [3.18]$$

Although the statistical distributions used in engineering are often Gaussian or uniform, they are not always like that. It is better to look for a family of polynomials that are orthogonal for the statistical distribution in use. However, if such family has no simple analytical expression or if the support of the real input distribution is not as in Table 3.1, then an isoprobabilistic transformation can be used.

Let us denote P the probability law governing a random variable X and $F_X(x)$ the PDF of the random variable X that is monotone and defined as [3.19]

$$F_X(x) = P[X \leq x] \qquad [3.19]$$

If Y is defined as $Y = F_X(X)$, then as [3.20] shows, Y has a uniform distribution.

$$F_Y(x) = P[Y \leq x] = [F_X(x) \leq x] = P\left[X \leq F_X^{-1}(x)\right] = F_X\left(F_X^{-1}(x)\right) = x \qquad [3.20]$$

Advanced transformations, such as the Nataf [NAT 62] or Rosenblatt [ROS 52] transforms, can be used to recast a problem having correlated components into a problem having non-correlated random variables.

The modal expansion [3.7] involves an infinite number of polynomials. For practical implementation, a finite dimensional PCE has to be built.

Let us denote $\hat{Y}$ a truncation of the generalized PCE.

$$\hat{Y} = \sum_{\alpha=0}^{P-1} \beta_\alpha \psi_\alpha(X) \qquad [3.21]$$

where P is the number of polynomials in the truncated series. The error ε between the infinite PCE and the finite one is given by [3.22]

$$Y - \hat{Y} = \varepsilon \qquad [3.22]$$

Depending on the input variables and on the maximal polynomial degree retained, the number of polynomials can be significant. Considering multivariate polynomials, ψ_k, having M input variables and assuming that N is the total maximum degree of them

$$\forall k \equiv \{k_i\},\ \sum_{i=1}^{M} k_i \leq N \qquad [3.23]$$

the size of this finite-dimensional basis is given by [3.24]

$$P = \binom{M+N}{N} = C_{N+M}^{N} = \frac{(N+M)!}{(N)!M!} \qquad [3.24]$$

The cardinal quickly becomes huge when the number of input variables M is greater than a few. It is affected by the so-called curse of dimensionality. For instance, if the model has four inputs and if we start with a polynomial order of 4, that is quite a simple problem since 70 coefficients will have to be calculated, the number of coefficients to estimate is 330 with a polynomial order of 7. Equation [3.21] provides the surrogate model $\hat{Y}$ we are looking for and that will be substituted to the FDTD calculations.

At this step, the validity of such a model arises fundamentally. Indeed, the use of alternative substitute models requires a method to validate these surrogate models. Among the existing methods for the assessment of a generalization aptitude of a model, the leave-one-out cross-validation (LOOCV) is often used in the domain of computer experimentation. Before discussing them, the first challenge is to obtain the generalized PCE coefficients.

3.5. Calculation of the PC coefficients

The mathematical framework of the generalized PCE is well defined and seems to be fitted for numerical dosimetry. The next step is the question of the assessment of the PCE coefficients. They can be estimated using spectral projections or least-square regressions.

3.5.1. *Coefficient assessment using spectral projection*

Spectral projection was first investigated in dosimetry [SIL 09] since this approach is often used in electromagnetism with modal decomposition, for instance with plane waves or spherical modes. With this approach, the orthogonality properties of the chaos polynomials are used to calculate the coefficients.

Assuming normalized polynomials (i.e. $||\psi_k|| = 1$) and Y the response of a physical model [3.6] to the random input $X(\omega)$, the coefficient β_m can be obtained using a projection [3.25] and [3.26] since the inner product of different polynomials is equal to zero [3.27]

$$\beta_m = \int \mathcal{M}(x)\,\psi_m(x) f_X(x)dx = \sum_{k=0}^{\infty}\left(\int \beta_k \psi_k(x)\,\psi_m(x) f_X(x)dx\right) \quad [3.25]$$

$$\beta_m = E[\mathcal{M}(X)\psi_m(X)] \quad [3.26]$$

$$\beta_m = \sum_{k=0}^{\infty}(\beta_k < \psi_k \psi_m >) = \sum_{k=0}^{\infty}(\beta_k \delta_{k,m}) \quad [3.27]$$

In case of numerical experiments, $\mathcal{M}(x)$ represents a complex response of a system, so the integral cannot be calculated in the close form. In this case, numerical integration techniques have to be used.

Numerical integration techniques are based on the integration weights, $w^{(i)}$, the random or deterministic integration nodes, $x^{(i)}$, and the number of estimations, L [3.28]. The accuracy of the estimation depends on the number and choice of the sampling.

$$\beta_m \approx \hat{\beta}_m = \sum_{i=1}^{L} w^{(i)} \mathcal{M}(x^{(i)}) \psi_m(x^{(i)}) \quad [3.28]$$

The simplest method to assess this is the MC method. In this case, the standard error, decrease in $1/\sqrt{L}$, induces a low convergence rate, which is a well-known drawback of MC simulations. The Latin hypercube sampling (LHS) and the quasi-random or low discrepancy sequences are more efficient than the Monte Carlo method (MCM) but the numerical integrations still need a large number of simulations. Moreover, these simulations have to be conducted for the expected coefficients and the number of these coefficients can be significant [3.24]. At the end, the overall number of simulations can be huge, which is often not compatible with the FDTD constraints.

Quadrature techniques provide alternative approaches for selecting the integration nodes and weights, but this approach is still affected by the so-called curse of dimensionality.

For multiple input variables, the basic method and the tensor product require the use of the L^M point, where M is the number of random input variables and L is the number of points used by 1D quadrature. In order to overcome this issue, sparse quadrature schemes using the Smolyak algorithm [SMO 63] that uses a multidimensional grid construction and sparse grids can be used to reduce the simulation effort. Advanced methods such as the Clenshaw–Curtis [CLE 60] formulation can reduce the number of collocation points (see Figure 3.3) even further.

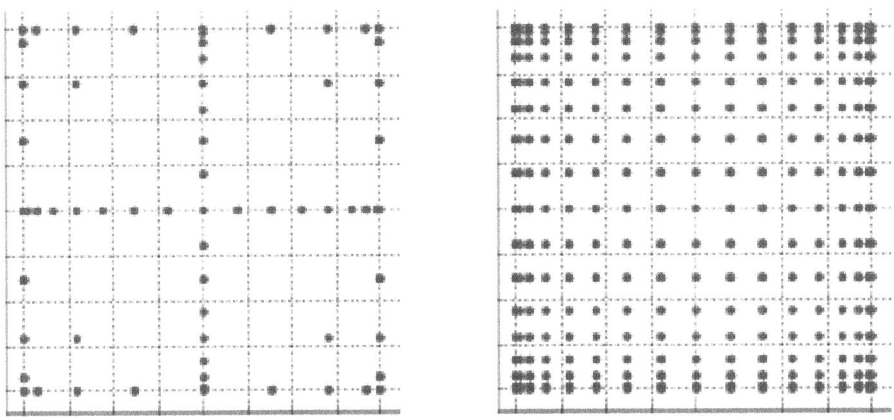

a) b)

Figure 3.3. *Collocation points with a) sparse grids and b) tensorial product*

In spite of these efforts, as shown in Table 3.2, the number of simulations needed is still significant even for advanced methods [CAR 08].

In conclusion, the quadrature approach combined with sparse grids can be used for problems involving a small number of variables. In practical problems, the number of inputs is often higher than 3 or 4 and in this case the projection approach is not really compatible with FDTD.

Order\number of input	1	2	3	4
1	3	5	7	9
2	5	13	25	41
3	9	29	69	137
4	17	65	177	401
5	33	145	441	1,105

Table 3.2. *Number of simulations versus order and number of uncertain variables for sparse grids*

3.5.2. *Coefficient assessment using regression*

Because of the significant effort required to assess the coefficients of the PC expansion with spectral projection, the calculation of these coefficients using least-square regression has been investigated. In this case, the strategy is to compute the coefficients that minimize the mean-square error of approximation of the model response. In engineering problems, the polynomial interpolation and linear regressions are often used to link the response of a system to explanatory variables and unknown functions. The calculation of the coefficients of the PCE took advantage of this existing knowledge.

Consider a model based on a truncation of the PCE [3.21] and also an observation vector, $y = \{y^{(1)}, y^{(2)}, \dots, y^{(m)}\}$, composed of the results of FDTD calculations (that are the "realizations"), performed at $x = \{x^{(1)}, x^{(2)}, \dots, x^{(m)}\}$ samples.

$$y^{(i)} = \sum_{\alpha=0}^{P-1} \beta_\alpha \psi_\alpha\left(x^{(i)}\right) + \varepsilon^{(i)} \qquad [3.29]$$

As described in [3.33], x can be a vector of M components.

Let us denote $z_{i,j} = \psi_j\left(x^{(i)}\right)$ the estimation of the polynomial (ψ_j) at the point $x^{(i)}$. $j \in [0, P-1]$. P is the number of polynomials involved in the truncation, and $i \in [1, m]$ represents the realizations.

The linear regression will look for a model such as [3.31]:

$$y = z\beta + \varepsilon \quad [3.30]$$

with the notation

$$z = \begin{bmatrix} z_{1,1} & .. & z_{1,P} \\ .. & z_{i,j} & .. \\ z_{m,1} & .. & z_{m,P} \end{bmatrix} z_{i,j} = \Psi_j(x^{(i)}) \quad [3.31]$$

and

$$\beta = \begin{bmatrix} \beta_1 \\ .. \\ \beta_P \end{bmatrix} \qquad y = \begin{bmatrix} y^{(1)} \\ .. \\ y^{(m)} \end{bmatrix} \qquad \varepsilon = \begin{bmatrix} \varepsilon^{(1)} \\ .. \\ \varepsilon^{(m)} \end{bmatrix} \quad [3.32]$$

The most common method used to assess β is the ordinary least square. This approach is conceptually simple, computationally straightforward and consists of minimization of the sum of squared residuals. This method provides a closed-form expression of $\hat{\beta}$ [3.33]:

$$\hat{\beta} = \{z^T z\}^{-1} z^T y \quad [3.33]$$

The estimation value of $\hat{\beta}$ is unbiased if the errors have finite variance and are uncorrelated with the explanatories variables (i.e. $E[z_i \varepsilon_i] = 0$)).

3.6. Design of experiments

This chapter will now focus on the design of experiments used to build the surrogate model. As explained in earlier chapters, the observation vector, $y = \{y^{(1)}, y^{(2)}, .., y^{(m)}\}$, is the result of FDTD calculations performed numerically on the $x = \{x^{(1)}, x^{(2)}, .., x^{(m)}\}$ samples.

As an example, in the case of a person exposed to an access point having variable angles of emission (θ, φ), the experimental design consists of selecting the "experiences" that are, in this case, a set of angles of emission

$\{(\theta_i, \varphi_i), \ldots, (\theta_j, \varphi_j), \ldots\}$ for which the whole-body SAR, for example, will be calculated.

To limit the computational "budget" (i.e. time and memory needed to carry out the simulations), the experiments must be optimally sampled to estimate model parameters. In case of physical experiments, repeat an operation that will induce some random local change and new results. In fact, in many of these laboratory experiments, it is assumed that the presence of random errors in the conditions of the experiment (e.g. position of the equipment, relative position of the probe) induces random errors in the measurement. This does not exist, hopefully, with deterministic numerical simulations. Indeed, repeating numerical experiments under the same conditions is not relevant since it does not provide any additional information and will only duplicate the result. The design of numerical experiments has to "mimic" the real world and organize the possible variations of the input according to their possible variations (e.g. Gaussian, uniform). The choice of the design of numerical experiments (e.g. position, posture and angle), where the simulations are conducted, is crucial and must meet several constraints.

First, the numerical experiments must be distributed in space as uniformly as possible in order to capture possible nonlinearities (relative to input variables) of the simulated phenomenon. At this stage, it is important to note that this uniformity is somewhat inconsistent with the need for a blind sampling to avoid bias.

Second, the initial input distribution (e.g. uniform) must subsist if a dimensionality reduction is performed. Indeed, when problems have a large dimension, that is to say that they have many input parameters, it is common to observe that the calculations depend heavily on only a few influential variables or on main components consisting of linear combinations of these variables. It is therefore important to keep the uniform filling property even in projection onto subspaces. The third constraint is linked to parsimony. This constraint is not fundamental from a theoretical point of view, but is the bottleneck of many practical situations. The number of simulations must be large enough to estimate all the coefficients of the approximate model but it must be limited to reduce the number of simulations to conduct. In the case of SAR calculations, for which computational times can be a few hours, the latter constraint is fundamental.

The design of experiments has been discussed in many textbooks and PhD reports [FRA 08]. One method to address the problem of filling the experimental area space is to select points on a regular grid. This approach can obviously lead to the wrong model by ignoring some features of the phenomenon due to the regular spacing. Dense meshing can help respond to the previous concern, but a regular dense filling will lead to a very large number of experiments and at the end heavy calculations that are not in line with parsimony. Such a limit can be solved using a random selection scheme.

In practice, such a completely random approach can create, as shown in Figure 3.4, a non-uniform sampling of the space that can lead to put too much weight on some part of the space, and therefore create a biased surrogate model.

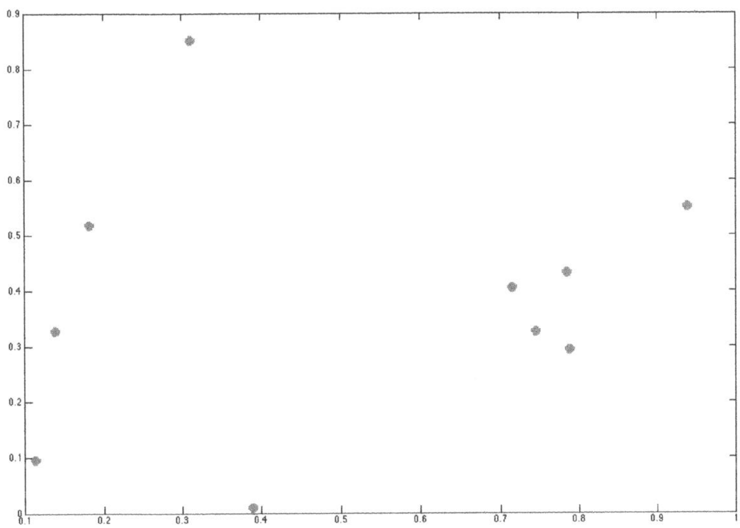

Figure 3.4. *Example of random non-uniform sampling of 10 points for two variables having uniform distributions*

The LHS [MCK 79] is, among the existing methods dedicated to the planning of experiments, a well-known statistical method. It generates a sample of a plausible set of parameter values from a multidimensional statistical distribution while taking care of a uniform filling of space. The principle of LHS is quite simple; Figure 3.5 shows a two-dimensional example. Consider an objective of N samples. A square grid is built based on equally probable N intervals of each dimension (in this example rows and columns). After that, one random sample in each row and each column is selected. This sampling is a Latin square sampling. The generalization of this simple concept to an arbitrary number of dimensions is known as "Latin hypercube sampling".

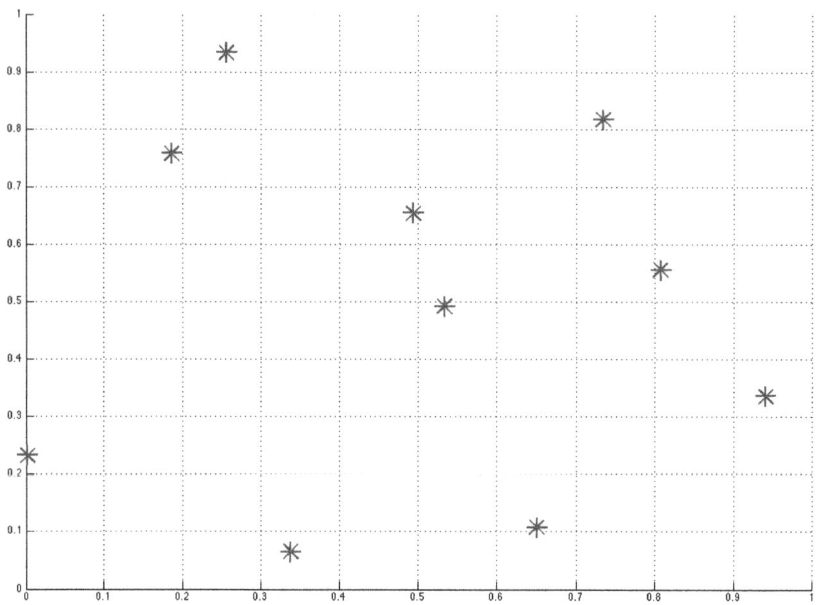

Figure 3.5. *LHS for M=10 points and two variables having uniform distribution*

The number of possible combinations of a LHS of M divisions and N variables is given by [3.34]:

$$\left(\prod_{p=0}^{M-1}(M-p)\right)^{N-1} = (M!)^{N-1} \quad [3.34]$$

The use of LHS does not prevent possible bad space filling. Figure 3.6 shows some possible two-dimensional combinations that do not fill the space uniformly.

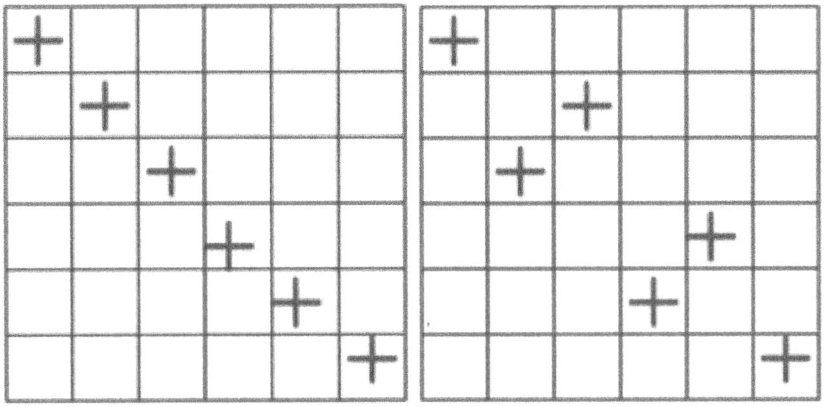

Figure 3.6. *Examples of LHS with N=2 (dimensions) and M=6 (intervals)*

A better space filling can be obtained using the "maxi–min" criteria. With this method, the LHS and the maximization of the distance between experiments are used together. The minimum Euclidean $d_{\min}^{(i)}$ distance between the points of the possible designs, $p^{(i)}$, of experiments can be calculated for all the possible experiment plans, $\{p^{(i)}\}$. The design of experiments having the maximum of the minimum distance, $d = \text{maxi}_i \left\{d_{\min}^{(i)}\right\}$, can be considered as the best plan from the space filling point of view.

In case of iterative approaches and minimization of calculations, it is often necessary to enlarge existing sampling plans. However, because of the heavy calculations, as they are in dosimetry, it is important to reuse the existing sampled points in a new planning.

The nested Latin hypercube sampling (NLHS), [WAN 03, QIA 09] allows us to add a point to an existing LHS. Let us consider an initial LHS designed for N variables and M samples. With a new point added to the M

initial samples, we can build a new LHS. Following the LHS rule, the range of each variable is divided into *M*+1 equally probable intervals and *M*+1 sample points should be placed in these intervals. The new intervals are by definition smaller than the initial ones (that have been designed for *M* samples), so all the existing points are located in different intervals of the new LHS. The NLHS will keep the existing point and only add a point to satisfy the Latin hypercube criteria (only one sample in each row and each column). NLHS provides a very good trade-off between randomness and parsimony.

3.7. Predictive model validation

The predictive ability of surrogate models that will replace the heavy simulation (FDTD in our case) needs to be checked and agreed. To check the accuracy assessment of a model, the first intuitive approach is to analyze the errors of the prediction. In statistical data analysis, the "variability" of the data set is measured through different sums of squares and in particular the total sum of squares (known as SST or TSS) and the residual sum of squares (known as RSS or SSR). SST and SSR are given by

$$\mathrm{SST} = \sum_i (y_i - \bar{y})^2 \qquad [3.35]$$

$$\mathrm{SSR} = \sum_i (y_i - \hat{y}_i)^2 \qquad [3.36]$$

In [3.35] and [3.36], $y^{(i)}$ and $\widehat{y^{(i)}}$ arc, respectively, the observed and predicted values, and $\bar{y}$ is the mean value given by [3.37]:

$$\bar{y} = \frac{1}{M}\sum_{i=1}^{M} y^{(i)} \qquad [3.37]$$

With regression, a coefficient of determination, R^2, is often used. This parameter is given by [3.38] and provides information about the goodness of fit of a model.

$$R^2 = \frac{\mathrm{SST}-\mathrm{SSR}}{\mathrm{SST}} \qquad [3.38]$$

R^2 criteria are well suited for the data analysis, but not really for the analysis of the predictive ability of a surrogate modeling. Indeed, having R^2 close to 1 does not provide information on the predictive aptitude of the model. Even if the predictions are bad, the overfitting or overtraining can leads us to have this coefficient close to one.

In the domain of design planning numerical experiments and surrogate model establishment, cross-validation is often used for the assessment of a predictive aptitude of a model. The qualification of a predictive model (e.g. surrogate model) is based, on the one hand, on a data set of known data on which the learning is performed and, on the other hand, another data set of known, but not used data, in learning and on which the model is tested.

Cross-validation defines a method for testing the quality of the model in its learning phase; while avoiding overfitting or overtraining, the ultimate goal is to provide an indicator of the quality prediction model.

Consider y_1 and $y_2 = \{y_2{}^{(1)}, y_2{}^{(2)}, .., y_2{}^{(m)}\}$ as two sets of, respectively, training and test data. The surrogate model, $\hat{y} = \widehat{\mathcal{M}}(\mathrm{x})$, is built using y_1 and will be tested using y_2. The performance of the model can be assessed through the mean square error (MSE), which measures the average of the squares of the "errors", that is the difference between the estimator and what is estimated.

With the present notation, the MSE, ε, is defined as

$$\varepsilon = \frac{1}{\mathrm{M}} \sum_{\mathrm{p}=1}^{\mathrm{M}} \left(\widehat{y_2{}^{(p)}} - y_2{}^{(p)}\right)^2 \qquad [3.39]$$

As explained in an earlier section, the simulations carried out in dosimetry can be cumbersome. In this case, the production of two data sets, the "training" and the "test", is not always possible or can require significant resources. LOOCV and the bootstrap methods can be used to the compute data as learning and testing each in turn. They are therefore well suited for the dosimetry context, for which parsimony is a key question.

LOOCV is a very intuitive method. Let us consider M experiments $\{\mathrm{y}^{(i)}\}_{i \in [1,M]}$, with $\mathrm{y}^{(i)} = \mathcal{M}(\mathrm{x}^{(i)})$. M–1 experiments can be used to build a model and the remaining experiment used to test the model. If we consider the M simulations, $y = \{y^{(1)}, y^{(2)}, .., y^{(m)}\}$, that have been performed and if we note $\widehat{\mathcal{M}_{-\mathrm{J}}}$ the model based on M–1 simulations, $\{y^{(1)}, y^{(2)}, .., y^{(M)}\} - \{y^{(j)}\}$, then we can estimate the MSE of the model using [3.40]

$$\varepsilon_{LOOCV} = \frac{1}{M}\sum_{i=1}^{M}\left((\widehat{\mathcal{M}(x^{(i)}}) - \mathcal{M}(x^{(i)})\right)^2 \qquad [3.40]$$

To help the interpretation of this error, we can calculate the coefficient of determination Q^2 from this error.

$$Q^2 = 1 - \frac{\varepsilon rr_{loo}}{\widehat{\sigma}_y^2} \qquad [3.41]$$

where $\widehat{\sigma}_y^2$ is the variance of the outputs Y. Having Q^2 close to 1 indicates a good generalization aptitude of the surrogate model.

The bootstrap approach is another simple and intuitive method [EFR 79] that does not require additional information other than that available in the sample. This approach is based on constructing a number of new samples (called bootstrap sample or re-samples) obtained by random sampling with replacement from the original sample and having the size of the observed dataset.

3.8. Surrogate modeling for dosimetry

3.8.1. *Surrogate modeling with full PCE basis*

The five steps for the construction of a surrogate model using the PC are described in the flowchart of Figure 3.7:

1) Identifying and characterizing the input variables. The accuracy of the overall process will depend on this, so this is a key step. In many cases, the knowledge about the inputs' statistical distribution is weak. The typical values and extreme values are known but the distribution is often unknown. In dosimetry, the "worst case" is the usual approach and the statistical distribution of the input is unknown. As an example, we can have some idea on the relative position of the phone close to the head but no studies have been carried out to characterize the distribution of the positioning angle.

2) Building the polynomial family relevant for the inputs and the characteristics of the inputs (e.g. Legendre polynomials if the inputs have uniform distribution). Isoprobabilist transformation can be used.

3) Building the experimental design (see section 3.6) taking into account the computational budget (e.g. a LHS), the number of inputs (given by the problem) and the degree of PCE. For example, with four inputs and a polynomial order of 4, as shown previously, we will need 70 coefficients. If we do not use an iterative process, the number of samplings, selected using LHS, has to be larger than 70 and large enough to avoid a bad conditioning of the information matrix of the least-square formulation.

4) Calculating the coefficients using a least-square regression [3.33] as described in section 3.5.2.

5) Checking the quality of the surrogate model using the LOOCV approach described in section 3.7.

After this:

i) if the accuracy is in line with the target accuracy, then the surrogate model is ready;

ii) otherwise new sample points have to complement (i.e. FDTD simulations have to be performed) the initial LHS until the quality reaches the target accuracy.

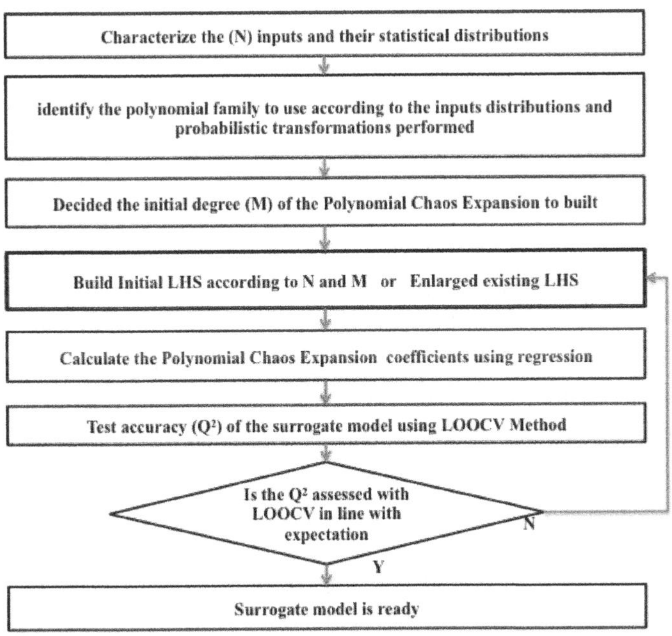

Figure 3.7. *Computational scheme of the surrogate built using full PCE*

This approach is quite straightforward but realistically impossible using all the polynomials involved in the polynomial basis if the polynomial order of the number of unknowns is significant. Indeed, such an approach needs a very large number of simulations that are not, most of the time, achievable in dosimetry. For instance, with a PCE using all the polynomials, the cardinal of the basis, with 5 input variables and a polynomial order up to 7 is 792. As shown in Figure 3.8, the number of polynomials can be huge; this constraint is known as the curse of dimensionality.

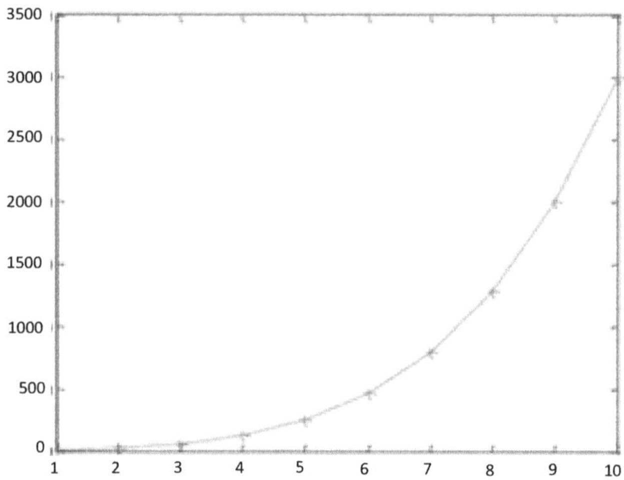

Figure 3.8. *Cardinal of the PCE basis with maximum order fifth versus the number of variables*

As we can expect, not all the polynomials have the same importance in the PCE truncation. Based on studies performed in the computational mechanics domain, sparse PCE basis [EFR 79] can be used to limit the computational effort. The following section will introduce sparse PC in stochastic dosimetry.

3.8.2. *Surrogate modeling with sparse PCE basis*

The polynomials involved in the truncation of the PCE may not have the same importance. Keeping constant the cardinal of the polynomials basis, the objective could be, as illustrated in Figure 3.9, the selection of the most important polynomials. For uncertainty propagation and SA, studies have been carried out [BLA 09] to set up a sparse PCE iteratively.

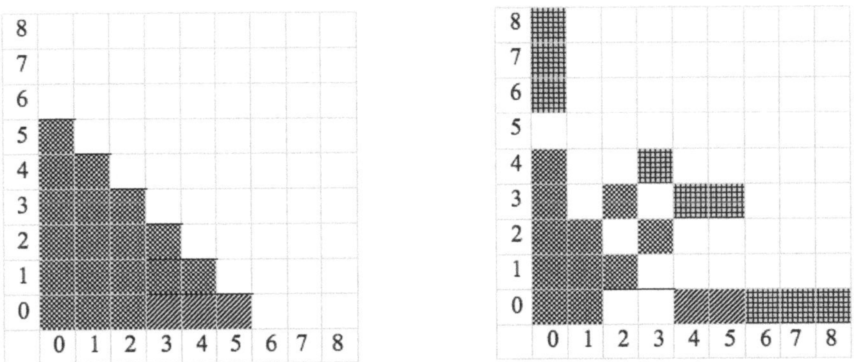

Figure 3.9. *Example of selection of polynomials keeping constant the cardinal of the polynomials basis*

Such a sparse basis can be built using different strategies. Within the mechanical domain, the use of the "sparsity-of-effects" principle, stating that the main effects and low-order interactions principally govern most models, has been investigated. Hyperbolic index sets have been used [BLA 11] to select the PC basis. This approach is quite easy to implement (select the polynomial having the global order below a hyperbolic curve) and seems to be relevant for mechanical problems but seems less relevant in electromagnetism and dosimetry.

In stochastic dosimetry, taking into account previous studies [BLA 11], the applicability of "LARS" methods to select a relevant PC basis has been investigated. The LARS method is a generic name for two kinds of method: on the one hand, the least angle regression (LAR) method [EFR 04], and on the other hand, the least absolute shrinkage and selection operator (LASSO) method [TIB 96].

LARS is objectively and significantly less easy to implement than the hyperbolic approach; LARS has proven [BLA 09, BLA 11, KER 14

ARY 12] its efficiency and its ability to handle engineering problems [BLA 11], including the electromagnetics problems as well as those encountered in bio-electromagnetism [WIA 15].

The idea governing LARS is to select, among a large set of polynomials forming a basis linked to a full truncation, the most influential polynomials. Toward this objective, LARS iteratively selects those polynomials having the greatest impact from the point of view of their correlation with the residual. With this method, the algorithm chooses, one by one, the polynomials in descending order of influence. This method provides many possible truncations having increasing sizes. Accordingly, in the flowchart described in Figure 3.7, the steps from "calculate the PCE coefficient using regression" linked to the computational scheme have to be replaced by a new one, shown in Figure 3.10, describing the process of selection of polynomials using LARS and selecting, using LOOCV, the best truncations.

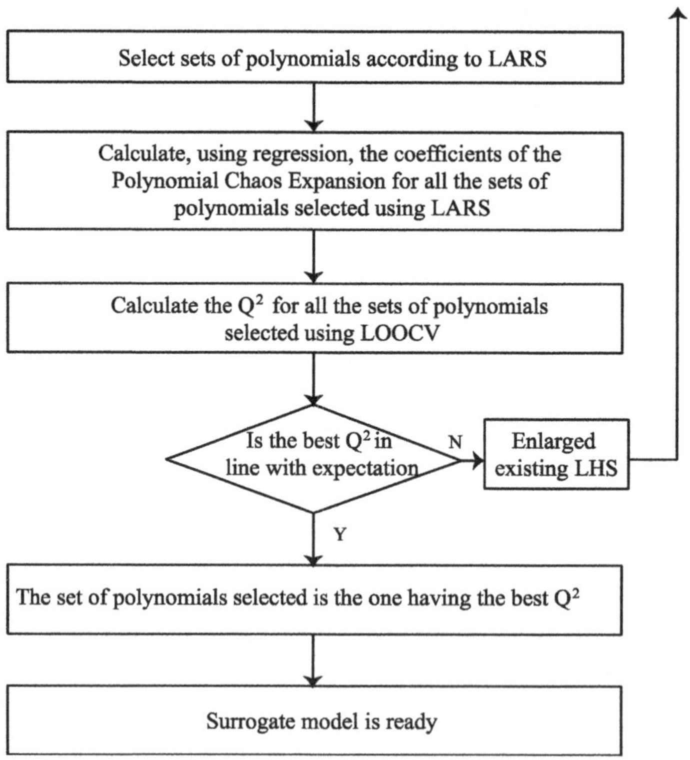

Figure 3.10. *Computational scheme of the surrogate built using sparse PCE*

3.8.3. *Stochastic dosimetry and SAR uncertainty linked to the phone position*

The technical standards (e.g. CENELEC or IEC) have defined two test positions (known as "cheek" and "tilt") to check the compliance of mobile phones with safety limits when the intended use of such equipment is close to the head. These configurations are used in a procedure that uses a homogeneous phantom (known as a Specific Anthropomorphic Mannequin (SAM)) designed to overestimate human exposure.

This methodology is useful and efficient to ensure compliance with exposure limits but obviously does not address the need, for the epidemiologists, of characterization of the distribution of the exposure associated with various uses of phones. The characterization of such real exposure requires us to investigate the impact on head exposure of variable phone positions. As explained in earlier sections, the usual approaches that use MC are not suitable for FDTD. In line with earlier section and to overcome this limitation, a sparse PCE has been used [GHA 13] to analyze the influence of variable phone usage on the maximum SAR over 10 g in the head (SAR10g) response. As illustrated in Figure 3.12, a handset phone is located close to the head of the Duke human phantom, part of the virtual family [CHR 10]. The handset model is a generic model composed of a print circuit board, a screen, a battery and a patch antenna located on the top of the phone model.

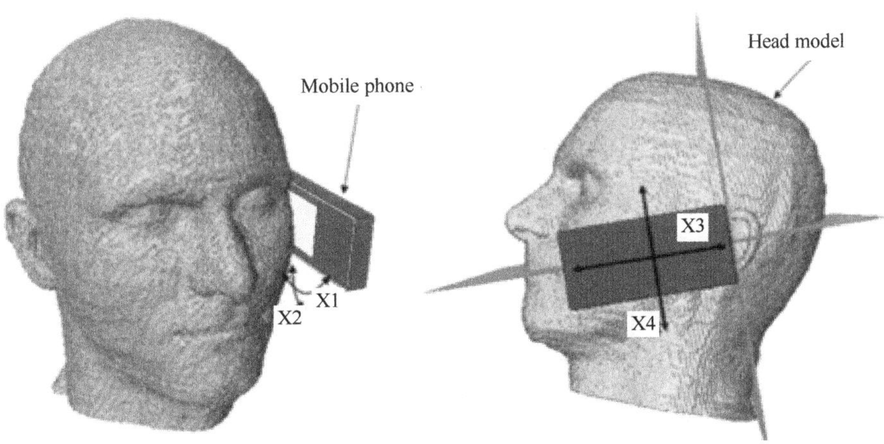

Figure 3.11. *Generic phone model located close to the head of the Duke human phantom*

Four parameters, X_1, X_2, X_3 and X_4, govern the rotation and translation of the phone model (see Figure 3.12) relative to the head. The support of the uniform distributions of these parameters are, respectively, [0°, 30°], [−15°, +15°], [5 mm, 30 mm], [−10 mm, +10 mm].

The procedure described previously has been used to build a SAR10 g surrogate model using a sparse approach. The initial experimental design was composed of M=25 points $\left\{\left(x_1^{(1)}, x_2^{(1)}, x_3^{(1)}, x_4^{(1)}\right), \ldots \left(x_1^{(i)}, x_2^{(i)}, x_3^{(i)}, x_4^{(i)}\right), \ldots\right\}$, selected using the LHS method. This experimental design has been, after that, enriched iteratively using a NLHS.

In this application, the input variables are uniform. The Legendre orthogonal polynomials are therefore suitable for the PCE. In this case, the support of the inputs must be $[-1, 1]$, so an iso-probabilist transform has to be used to link X_1, X_2, X_3, X_4 and the standardized PCE Legendre polynomial inputs.

The sparse PCE has been obtained using on the one hand the hyperbolic index sets and on the other hand LARS. For the hyperbolic approach, as illustrated in Table 3.3, the sparse PCE surrogate model produced by the iterative procedure allows us to have, for an accuracy of 10^{-2} (assessed using a LOOCV), a PCE of degree p = 8, which contains only 18 terms instead of the 495 terms that can be requested by the usual full PCE according to [3.34].

PCE order	Number of significant polynomials	Number of simulations	Q^2
p=2	7	30	0.9
p=5	9	43	0.95
p=8	18	88	0.99
p=12	29	122	0.999

Table 3.3. *Order of PCE polynomials, number of simulations and Q^2 of the sparse SAR10 g surrogate PCE model obtained with the iterative process and the "hyperbolic" index set*

As explained previously, LARS is much more efficient than other sparse approaches. In the present example, a LOOCV $(1 - Q^2)$ accuracy of 1% is obtained with a seventh order and 71 simulations (15 significant polynomial coefficients to compare with the 330 that are requested using a full PCE).

The 0.1% is obtained with 103 simulations (i.e. 78 simulations added iteratively to the 25 initial ones using the NLHS); in this case, 27 polynomials are involved in the surrogate model. Figure 3.12 shows the probability distribution function (PDF) of 122 simulations that have been performed.

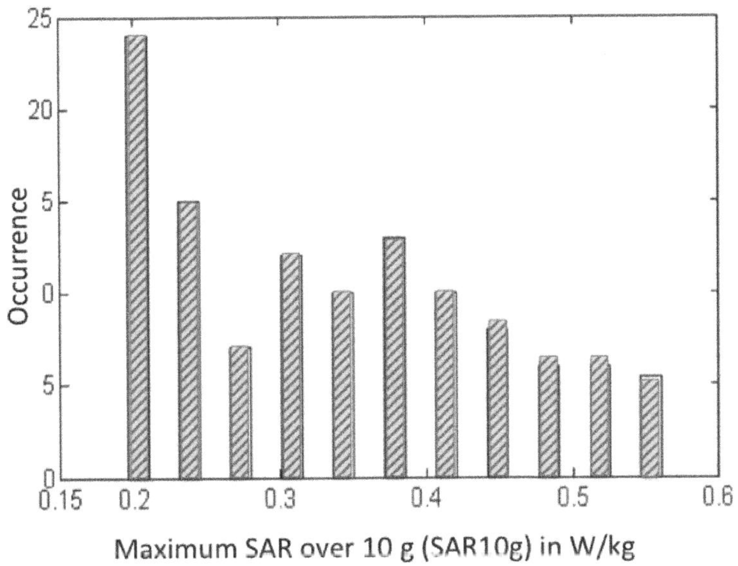

Figure 3.12. *Distribution of the 122 FDTD simulations that have been performed*

Figure 3.13 provides the PDF of the FDTD simulations that have been performed but even if the experimental design has been done with LHS, the resulting PDF is not necessarily fully representative of that of the SAR10g linked to the variations of the position of the phone model relative to the head.

To assess this statistical distribution, we can use the SAR10g surrogate model that has been built and the MC approach to generate large number of outputs. Figure 3.14 shows the PDF of the SAR10g estimated using the surrogate models based on "full" PCE (order 3), sparse PCE using the hyperbolic index set and the sparse PCE built using LARS and 10,000 points $\left(x_1^{(i)}, x_2^{(i)}, x_3^{(i)}, x_4^{(i)}\right)$ selected using the usual MC process.

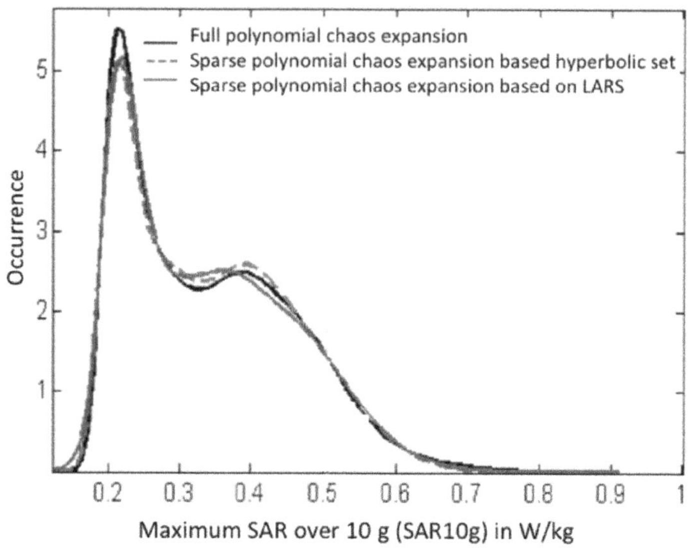

Figure 3.13. *PDF of the SAR10g based on different surrogate models ("full" PCE, sparse "hyperbolic" PCE and sparse LARS PCE) and 10,000 positions of the phone model relative to the head. For a color version of the figure, see www.iste.co.uk/wiart/radiofrequency.zip*

3.9. SA and signature of the PC

3.9.1. *SA and Sobol indices*

The SA investigates the apportionment in the output uncertainty (of a mathematical model or system) of the different sources of uncertainty of the inputs. SA is often divided into local and global SA. The influence, in the vicinity of given values, on the outputs of little variations of the inputs is addressed by local SA. Global SA studies and quantifies the output uncertainties linked to changes in the inputs over their domains of variation.

Different methods exist [SAL 00] to perform SA, among them the variance-based methods, also known as analysis of variance (ANOVA) with "Sobol's" decomposition [SOB 93], are often used. They are applicable for independent variables but methods exist for dependent variables [KUC 12]. With the ANOVA approach, the response $Y = \mathcal{M}(X)$ of a system having finite variance and independent inputs is divided [EFR 81] into main effects and interactions.

The response variance $D = \mathrm{Var}[Y]$ can be divided into partial variances

$$D_i = \mathrm{Var}_{X_i}\left[E[Y|X_i = x_i]\right] \qquad [3.42]$$

$$D_{i,j} = \mathrm{Var}_{X_i}\left[E\left[Y|X_i = x_i, X_j = x_j\right]\right] - D_i - D_j \qquad [3.43]$$

$$D_{i,j,k} = \mathrm{Var}_{X_i}\left[E\left[Y|X_i = x_i, X_j = x_j, X_k = x_k\right]\right] \\ -D_{i,j} - D_{i,k} - D_{j,k} - D_i - D_j - D_k \qquad [3.44]$$

where $E[Y|X_i = x_i]$ is the mean model response when the *i*th input parameter is kept fixed at a given value x_i; the variance of the latter is greater since this conditional mean varies as much as a function of x_i. The partial variance D_i measures the contribution of X_i, alone, to the uncertainty (variance) in Y (averaged over variations in other variables). Sobol's indices that are known to be good descriptors of the sensitivity of the model response to its input parameters, since they do not suppose any kind of linearity of the model, are defined as

$$S_{i_1,..i_s} = \frac{D_{i_1,..i_s}}{D} \qquad [3.45]$$

Sobol's indices are usually assessed using MC simulation that is not easy to carry out in the case of heavy calculation. The use of surrogate models alleviates the procedure. In the case of PCE, the calculations are greatly reduced since the knowledge of the coefficients of PCE allows for Sobol's indices without further calculation. Indeed, because of the orthonormality of the polynomials involved in the PCE, the total and partial variances can be assessed using the total or partial sums of the squared coefficients. With the same notation as in [3.29], the total variance is given by:

$$\widehat{D} = \mathrm{Var}(\widehat{Y}) = \sum_{k=0}^{P-1} \beta_k^2 \qquad [3.46]$$

The partial variances are given by

$$\widehat{D}_{i_1,\dots i_s} = \sum_{\alpha \in \mathcal{T}_{i_1,\dots i_s}} \beta_\alpha^2 \qquad [3.47]$$

where

$$\mathcal{T}_{i_1,\dots i_s} = \{\alpha\colon \alpha_k > 0, k \in (i_1, \dots i_s)\} \qquad [3.48]$$

Equation [3.48] shows that the partial variance $\widehat{D}_{i_1,\dots i_s}$ is obtained by summing up the squared coefficients of the relative polynomials that depend only on x_i.

$$S_{i_1,\dots i_s} = \frac{\sum_{\alpha \in \mathcal{T}_{i_1,\dots i_s}} \beta_\alpha^2}{\sum_{k=0}^{N-1} \beta_k^2} \qquad [3.49]$$

The total sensitivity indices S_i^T have also been defined to quantify the total effect of an input parameter onto the output. They are defined from the sum of all partial sensitivity indices $S_{i_1,\dots i_s}$ involving parameter i.

$$S_i^T = 1 - \frac{\widehat{D}_{-i}}{\widehat{D}} \qquad [3.50]$$

where $\widehat{D}_{-i}$ is the sum of all $\widehat{D}_{i_1,\dots i_s}$ that do not include index i.

3.9.2. *Sensitivity of SAR linked to the phone position*

The coefficients estimated in the previous section can be used to perform the SA of the head exposure with respect to the four parameters, X_1, X_2, X_3, X_4, governing the rotation and translation of the phone model relative to the head (see Figure 3.14).

Figure 3.15 shows Sobol's indices estimated using the PCE coefficients. These indices show that the four most important parameters are S1, S3, S12 and S13. The total sensitivity indices have also been estimated.

The most important are S_1^T and S_3^T, which are, respectively, about 85% and 10%. The less important are S_4^T and S_2^T, which contribute less than 5% together. This analysis shows that the most important parameter is the rotation in the plane composed of the ears and mouth.

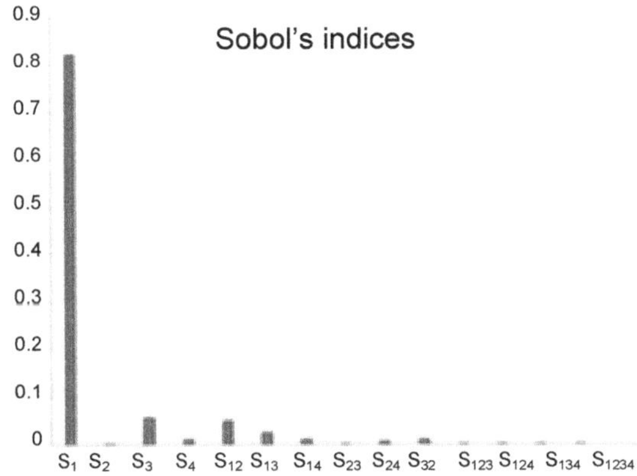

Figure 3.14. *Sobol's indices estimated using the PCE coefficients*

3.9.3. *PC signature*

In electromagnetism, the modal decomposition of electromagnetics is often used to study systems. Taking advantage of Parseval's theorem, the distribution of the energy over the modes is studied through a signature. As in such modal analysis, it is of interest to analyze the signature of the polynomial expansion (i.e. the coefficient affecting the polynomial).

The signature of the PC provides valuable information on the importance of the polynomials involved in the polynomial expansion and on the combination of the inputs involved in these influential polynomials. Such analysis has been carried out to study the variation in the field scattered by building façades. A numerical method based on Green's functions of semi-infinite medium was proposed in an initial study [MOS 10]; this method is fast but not enough to perform the large number of simulations required in a statistical study. To overcome this limitation, the PCE has been used to analyze the EMF field scattered by building façades [CER 14]. Compared with a MC approach, the number of required input samples has been reduced by more than one order of magnitude for the same precision in output distribution.

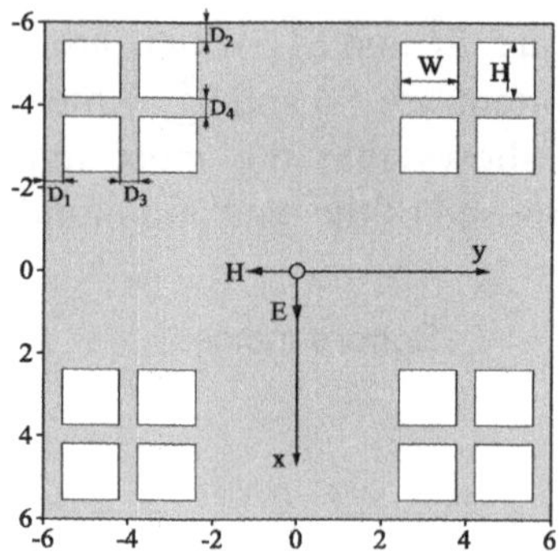

Figure 3.15. *Building façade model used in the stochastic analysis [MOS 10, KER 14]*

The problem has eight input variables: height and width of the windows and façade, separation distances between windows and between window and façade edges. Figure 3.15 shows the configuration. Uniform distribution and NLHS have been used in this study [KER 14]. Figure 3.16 shows the signature of the PCE composed of the coefficient values for all the polynomials involved in the PCE. The PCE's signature helps to identify the most important polynomial and is therefore a valuable complement to SA.

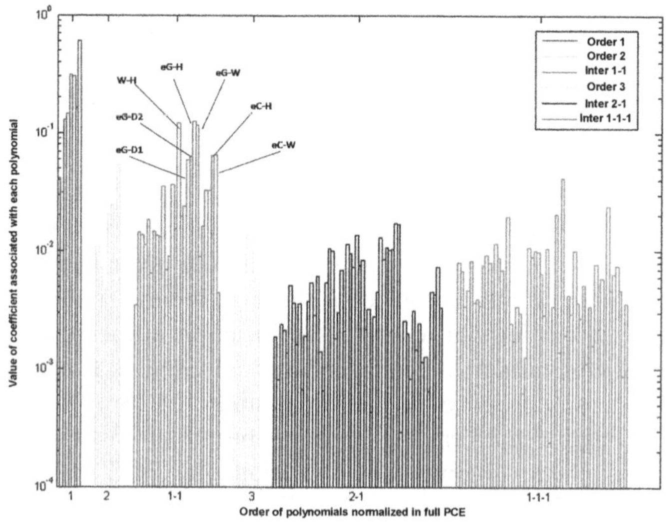

Figure 3.16. *Coefficient values for all the polynomials involved in the full PCE. For a color version of the figure, see www.iste.co.uk/wiart/radiofrequency.zip*

3.10. Parsimonious quintile estimation

Given the fact that, on the one hand, a numerical dosimetry simulation is expensive in terms of computational load and time, and, on the other hand, its preparation could also be complex and time consuming, studies have been carried out to propose a sequential sampling strategy where each computer trial is selected in order to estimate a quantile as accurately as possible by performing as few evaluations of the SAR as possible. The study, on the one hand, analyzed the problem with the Gaussian process [JAL 14] and, on the other hand, combined [KER 15] the PC and the Kriging approach.

3.11. Conclusion

The significant advances observed in the computational domain and in the area of numerical simulations, both from the standpoint of hardware and software, allow us today to envisage simulations considered impossible or at least inaccessible 15 years ago. As a result, numerical simulations are nowadays more and more used to design systems and estimate quantities such as antenna performances and SAR in the case of wireless communication systems.

Despite this progress, computational times are still a limit to performing SA and to monitoring and quantifying the impact on the outputs of simulations of possible variations of the inputs.

As described in this chapter, the statistical tools and in particular the PCE and the Kriging are mature methods to be used in electromagnetism and, in particular, numerical dosimetry to estimate and monitor the influence on exposure of uncertainties in geometrical and physical properties of a physical problem.

By adding a statistical dimension to a deterministic calculation and using the techniques of the propagation of uncertainties in a complex scenario, the electromagnetic fields and SAR distribution (or other outputs of simulations) can be presented by a confidence interval that makes the result more useful for subsequent decision-making.

Conclusion

> *"The difficult is that which can be done immediately; the impossible that which takes a little longer".*
>
> George SANTAYANA

As explained in the introduction to Chapter 1, wireless communication has a key impact on our present life and will play an important role in our daily life in the future. Because of the risk perception and concern about electromagnetic field (EMF), the dosimetry has become an important domain of applied electromagnetism with large interactions with antennas, telecommunications, epidemiology, biology and EMC.

The studies performed in the 1990s and in the 2000s have allowed us, using experimental and numerical techniques, to design methods dedicated to the compliance test of wireless systems and measurement of the exposure. With the improvement of computers and high-performance calculations, numerical dosimetry has been used more and more. The efficiency, aptitude and usability of methods such as finite difference in time domain (FDTD) have been significantly improved.

Much research effort has been carried out to create realistic human phantoms. Today, the design of wireless systems is performed using numerical methods to assess the SAR. Biological and epidemiological studies are also using FDTD to assess the exposure and design experiments.

Currently, dosimetry is facing the challenges of, on the one hand, the increasing complexity of networks and the increasing use of reconfigurable ones and of self-organizing ones, and, on the other hand, the versatile use of wireless systems with which the dosimetry methods also have to cope.

To characterize such variable exposure, the usual dosimetric numerical methods (e.g. FDTD) can require a very large number of simulations. In spite of the progress observed during recent decades in high-performance calculation, the deterministic approach is no longer applicable and a new age has started with stochastic dosimetry.

With the increasing use of the Internet of Things (IoT), mobile connections and traffic, human exposure assessment will use more and more statistical methods and models combining the deterministic numerical method, stochastic geometry, geostatistical tools and surrogate modeling. The new professors of Telecom ParisTech will have a key role in the combination of these different approaches within stochastic dosimetry.

Bibliography

[ABR 72] ABRAMOWITZ M., STEGUN I.A., *Handbook of Mathematical Functions with Formulas, Graphs, and Mathematical Tables*, 9th ed., Dover, New York, 1972.

[ACK 95] ACKERMAN, "Accessing the visible human project", D-Lib Magazine, available at: www.nlm.nih.gov/research/visible/visible_human.html, 1995.

[ADA 04] ADANE Y., WONG M.F., GATI A. *et al.*, "Accurate fast modeling for real base station antennas using gain patterns via spherical modes", *International Journal of Applied Electromagnetics and Mechanics*, vol. 19, no. 1, pp. 545–549, 2004.

[ADO 03] ADONIS P., Analyse dosimétrique des systèmes de téléphonie mobile de troisième génération, available at: http://adonis.telecom-paristech.fr, 2003.

[ALT 02] ALTMAN Z., BEGASSE B., DALE C. *et al.*, "Efficient models for base station antennas for human exposure assessment", *IEEE Transactions on Electromagnetic Compatibility*, vol. 44, no. 4, pp. 588–592, 2002.

[ANQ 09] ANQUEZ J., Modélisation de la femme enceinte à partir d'images 3D ultrasonores *et* IRM anténatales, pour l'étude de la dosimétrie, PhD Thesis, Télécom ParisTech, 2009.

[ARY 15] ARYA R.K., KERSAUDY P., WIART J. *et al.*, "Statistical analysis of periodic structures and frequency selective surfaces using the polynomial chaos expansions", *Forum for Electromagnetic Research Methods and Application Technologies*, vol. 12, November–December 2015.

[BAR 79] BARBER P.W., GANDHI, O.P., HAGMANN, M.J. *et al.*, "Electromagnetic absorption in a multilayered model of man", *IEEE Transactions on Biomedical Engineering*, vol. 26, no. 7, pp. 400–405, 1979.

[BEA 06] BEARD B.B, KAINZ W., ONISHI T., "Comparisons of computed mobile phone induced SAR in the SAM phantom to that in anatomically correct models of the human head", *IEEE Transactions on Electromagnetic Compatibility*, vol. 48, no. 2, 2006.

[BEA 08] BEARD *et al.*, KUSTER. *et al.*, WIART *et al.*, 2008.

[BER 00] BERENGER J.P., "A multiwire formalism for the FDTD method", *IEEE Transactions on Electromagnetic Compatibility*, vol. 42, no. 3, pp. 257–264, 2000.

[BER 94] BERENGER J.P., "A perfectly matched layer for the absorption of electromagnet waves", *Journal of Computational Physics*, vol. 114, pp. 185–200, 1994.

[BER 06] BERENGER J.P., "A Huygens subgridding for the FDTD method", *IEEE Transactionson Antennas Propagation*, vol. 54, pp. 3797–3804, 2006.

[BIB 10] BIBIN L., ANQUEZ J., DE LA PLATA ALCALDE J.P. *et al.*, "Whole body pregnant woman modeling by digital geometry processing with detailed utero-fetal unit based on medical images", *IEEE Transactions on Biomedical Engineering*, vol. 57, no. 10, pp. 2346–2358, 2010.

[BLA 09] BLATMAN G., Adaptive sparse polynomial chaos expansions for uncertainty propagation and sensitivity analysis, PhD Thesis, University Blaise Pascal Clermont Ferrand, 2009.

[BLA 11] BLATMAN G., SUDRET B. "Adaptive sparse polynomial chaos expansion based on least angle regression", *Journal of Computational Physics*, vol. 230, no. 6, pp. 2345–2367, 2011.

[BON 02] BONILLA M., WONG M.-F., HANNA V.F., "A finite-element formulation for FDTD-subgridding", *Microwave and Optical Technology Letters*, vol. 32, no. 2, 2002.

[BON 07] BONILLA M., ALQUIE G., FOUAD H.H. *et al.*, "A 3D FDTD-subgridding scheme derived from a finite element formulation", *Electromagnetics*, vol. 22, pp. 429–442, 2007.

[BRE 09] BRECKENKAMP J. *et al.*, "Feasibility of a cohort study on health risks caused by occupational exposure to radiofrequency electromagnetic fields", *Environmental Health*, vol. 29, pp. 8–23, 2009.

[BRE 89] BRETONES A.R., MARTIN R.G., SALINA SA., "DOGTIGI, a time-domain numerical code for the study of the interaction of electromagnetic pulses with thin-wire structures", *COMPEL*, vol. 8, no. l, pp. 39–61, 1989.

[BRE 98] BRETONES A.R., MITTRA R., MARTIN R.G., "A hybrid technique combining the method of moments in the time domain and FDTD", *IEEE Microwave and Guided Wave Letters*, vol. 8, no. 8, pp. 281–283, 1998.

[BRI 01] BRISHOUAL M., DALE C., WIART J. *et al.*, "Comparison of interpolation and extrapolation methods with a method using multiresolution wavelet transform in dosimetric experiments", *Annales des Télécommunications*, vol. 56, nos. 5–6, pp. 363–371, 2001.

[BRI 08] BRISHOUAL M., DALE C., WIART J. *et al.*, "Methodology to interpolate and extrapolate SAR measurements in a volume in dosimetric experiments", *IEEE Transactions on Electromagnetic Compatibility*, vol. 43, no. 3, pp. 382–389, 2008.

[BSI 01] BRITISH STANDARDS, Product standard to demonstrate the compliance of mobile phones with the basic restrictions related to human exposure to electromagnetic fields (300 MHz - 3 GHz), EN50360:2001, 2001.

[BSI 06] BRITISH STANDARDS, Human exposure to radio frequency fields from hand-held and body-mounted wireless communication devices. Human models, instrumentation, and procedures. Procedure to determine the specific absorption rate (SAR) for hand-held devices used in close proximity to the ear (frequency range of 300 MHz to 3 GHz), EN62209-1:2006, 2006.

[BSI 08] BRITISH STANDARDS, Basic standard for the in-situ measurement of electromagnetic field strength related to human exposure in the vicinity of base stations, EN50492, 2008.

[BUR 04] BURGUET J., GADI N., BLOCH I., "Realistic models of children heads from 3D MRI segmentation and tetrahedral mesh construction", *2nd International Symposium on 3D Data Processing, Visualization and Transmission*, Thessaloniki, Greece, pp. 631–638, 2004.

[CAM 47] CAMERON R.H., MARTIN WT., "The orthogonal development of nonlinear functionals in series of Fourier-Hermite functionals", *Annals of Mathematics*, vol. 2, no. 48, pp. 385–392, 1947.

[CAR 08] CARETTE-SILLY J., Modélisation avancée de l'absorption des ondes électromagnétiques dans les tissus biologiques, PhD Thesis, Université UPMC, 2008.

[CAR 10] CARDIS E., DELTOUR I., VRIJHEID M. *et al.*, "Brain tumour risk in relation to mobile telephone use: results of the INTERPHONE international case–control study", *International Journal of Epidemiology*, vol. 39, no. 3, pp. 675–694, 2010.

[CAS 13] CASSOLA V.F., KRAMER R., DE MELO LIMA V.J. *et al.* "Development of newborn and 1-year-old reference phantoms based on polygon mesh surfaces", *Journalof Radiological Protection,* vol. 33, no. 3, pp. 669–691, 2013.

[CHA 06] CHAUVIÈRE C., HESTHAVEN J.S., LURATI L., "Computational Modeling of uncertainty in time-domain electromagnetics", *SIAM Journal on Scientific Computing*, vol. 28, pp. 751–775, 2006.

[CHA 99] CHAILLOU S., WIART J., TABBARA W., "A subgridding scheme based on mesh nesting for the FDTD method", *Microwave and Optical Technology Letters*, vol. 22, no. 3, pp. 211–214, 1999.

[CHE 94] CHEW W.C., WEEDON W.H., "A 3D perfectly matched medium from modified Maxwell's equations with stretched coordinates", *Microwave and Optical Technology Letters*, vol. 7, no. 13, pp. 599–604, 1994.

[CHE 97] CHEVALIER M.W., LUEBBERS R.J., "FDTD local grids with materials traverse", *IEEE Transactions on Antennas Propagation*, vol. 45, pp. 411–421, 1997.

[CHR 10] CHRIST A., KAINZ W., HAHN. *et al.*, "The virtual family – development of surface-based anatomical models of two adults and two children for dosimetric simulations", *Physics in Medicine and Biology*, vol. 55, no. 2, pp. N23–N38, 2010.

[CIS 15] CISCO, Cisco Visual Networking Index: Global Mobile Data Traffic Forecast Update, 2014–2019, White Paper, 2015.

[CLE 60] CLENSHA W.C., CURTIS A.R., "A method for numerical integration on an automatic computer", *Numerical Mathematics*, vol. 2, pp. 197–205, 1960.

[CON 08] CONIL E., HADJEM A., LACROUX F. *et al.* "Variability analysis of SAR from 20 MHz to 2.4 GHz for different adult and child models using finite-difference time-domain", *Physics in Medicine and Biology*, vol. 53, pp. 1511–1525, 2008.

[CON 11] CONIL E., HADJEM A., GATI A. *et al.*, "Influence of plane wave incidence angle on whole body and local exposure at 2100 MHz", *IEEE Transactions on Electromagnetic Compatibility*, vol. 53, no. 1, pp. 48–52, 2011.

[COS 09] COSTEN F., BERENGER J.P., BROWN A.K., "Comparison of FDTD hard source with FDTD soft source and accuracy assessment in Debye Media", *IEEE Transactions on Antenna and Propagation,* vol. 57, no. 7, pp. 2014–2022, 2009.

[COU 28] COURANT R., FREIDRICHS K., LEWY H., "Uber diepartillenen differenzenglei chungen der mathematischen physik ", *Mathematische Annalen,* vol. 100, pp. 32–74, 1928.

[COV 91] COVER T.M., THOMAS J.A., *Elements of Information Theory*, Wiley, New York, 1991.

[CRI 80] CRISTY M., *Mathematical Phantoms Representing Children of Various Ages for Use in Estimates of Internal Dose*, Oak Ridge National Laboratory, Oak Ridge, TN, 1980.

[DAH 14] DAHDOUH, *et al.*, "A comprehensive tool for image-based generation of fe*t*us and pregnant women mesh models for numerical dosim*et*ry studies", *Physics in Medicine and Biology,* vol. 59, pp. 4583–4602, 2014.

[DEH 00] DEHAYES S., Prédiction et analyse des perturbations subies par un dispositif électronique placé dans un environnement électromagnétique sévère. Application à l'immunité des systèmes de communication, PhD Thesis, University of Paris VI, 2000.

[DEV 92] DEVEZE T., "Contribution à l'analyse, par différences finies, des équations de Maxwell dans le domaine temps", Thesis, Pierre and Marie Curie University Paris, 1992.

[DIM 05] DIMBYLOW P.J., "Development of the female voxel phantom, NAOMI and its application to calculations of induced current densities and electric fields from applied low frequency magnetic and electric fields", *Physics in Medicine and Biology*, vol. 50, no. 6, pp. 1047–1070, 2005.

[DIM 06] DIMBYLOW P.J., "Development of pregnant female, hybrid voxel-mathematical models and their application to the dosim*et*ry of applied magnetic and electric fields at 50 Hz", *Physics in Medicine and Biology,* vol. 51, no. 10, pp. 2383–2394, 2006.

[DIM 94] DIMBYLOW P.J., MANN S.M., "SAR calculations in an anatomically realistic model of the head for mobile communication transceivers at 900 MHz and 1.8 GHz", *Physics in Medicine and Biology*, vol. 39, pp. 1537–1553, 1994.

[DIM 97] DIMBYLOW P.J., "FDTD calculations of the whole-body averaged SAR in an anatomically realistic voxel model of the human body from 1 MHz to 1 GHz", *Physics in Medicine and Biology*, vol. 42, pp. 479–490, 1997.

[DIR 14] DIRECTIVE 2014/53/EU OF THE EUROPEAN PARLIAMENT AND OF THE COUNCIL, On the harmonisation of the laws of the Member States relating to the making available on the market of radio equipment and repealing Directive 1999/5/EC, 2014.

[DIR 16] DIRECTIVE RADIO AND TELECOMMUNICATIONS TERMINAL EQUIPMENT (R&TTE), available at http://ec.europa.eu/enterprise/sectors/rtte/index_en.htm, 2016.

[DRO 00] DROSSOS A., SANTOMAA V., KUSTER N., "The dependence of electro-magnetic energy absorption upon human head tissue composition in the frequency range of 300–3000 MHz", *IEEE Transactionson MicrowaveTheory Techniques*, vol. 48, no. 11, pp. 1988–1995, 2000.

[DUD 95] DUDLEY D.G., "Dyadic Green's funtions", in CHEW W.C. (ed.), *Waves and Fields in Inhomogeneous Media*, Wiley–IEEE Press, 1995.

[ECR 99] EUROPEAN COUNCIL RECOMMENDATION, The limitation of exposure of the general public to electromagnetic fields (0 Hz to 300 GHz) 1999/519/CE, 1999.

[EDE 03] EDELVIK F., "A new technique for accurate and stable modeling of arbitrarily oriented thin wires in the FDTD method", *IEEE Transactions on Electromagnetic Compatibility*, vol. 45, no. 2, pp. 416–423, 2003.

[EFR 04] EFRON B., HASTIE T., JOHNSTONE I. *et al.*, "Least angle regression", *Annals of Statistics*, vol. 32, pp. 407–499, 2004.

[EFR 79] EFRON B., "Bootstrap methods: another look at the Jackknife", *Annals of Statistics*, vol. 7, no. 1, pp. 1–2, 1979.

[EFR 81] EFRON B., STEIN C., "The Jacknife estimate of variance", *Annals of Statistics*, vol. 9, no. 3, pp. 586–596, 1981.

[EL 10] EL HABACHI A., CONIL E., HADJEM A. *et al.*, "Statistical analysis of whole-body absorption depending on anatomical human characteristics at a frequency of 2.1 GHz", *Physics in Medicine and Biology*, vol. 55, pp. 1875–1887, 2010.

[EUR 10] EUROPEAN COMMISSION, Electromagnetic Field Report, Special Europbarometer 347, Wave 73.3, 2010.

[FAR 00] FARAONE A., *et al.*, "Estimation of the average power density in the vicinity of cellular base-station collinear array antenna", *Vehicular Technology, IEEE Transactions*, vol. 49, no. 3, pp 984–996, 2000.

[FAR 94] FARKAS L.G., *Antropometry of the Head and Face*, Raven Press, New York, 1994.

[FIS 66] FISHER H.L., SNYDER W.S., "Annual progress report for period ending July 31 1966, Health Physics Division", Oak Ridge National Laboratory, Oak Ridge TN, 1966.

[FRA 08] FRANCO J., Planification d'expériences numériques en phase exploratoire pour la simulation des phénomènes complexes, PhD Thesis, Ecole Nationale Supérieure des Mines de Saint-Etienne, 2008.

[GAB 96a] GABRIEL S., LAU R.W., GABRIEL C., "The dielectric properties of biological tissues: II. Measurements in the frequency range 10 Hz to 20 GHz", *Physics in Medicine and Biology*, vol. 41, pp. 2251–2269, 1996.

[GAB 96b] GABRIEL S., LAU R.W., GABRIEL C., "The dielectric properties of biological tissues: III. Parametric models for the dielectric spectrum of tissues", *Physics in Medicinal* Biology, vol. 41, pp. 2271–2293, 1996.

[GAB 96c] GABRIEL C., GABRIEL S., CORTHOUT E., "The dielectric properties of biological tissues: I. Literature survey", *Physics in Medicinal Biology*, vol. 41 pp. 2231–2249, 1996.

[GAB 10] GABRIEL C., PEYMAN A., "Cole–cole parameters for the dielectric properties of porcine tissues as a function of age at microwave frequencies", *Physics in Medicine and Biology*, vol. 55, no. 15, pp. 413–419, 2010.

[GAJ 13] GAJŠEK P., RAVAZZANI J., WIART J. *et al.*, "Electromagnetic field (EMF) exposure assessment in Europe: radio frequency fields (10 MHz–6 GHz)", *Journal of Exposure Science and Environmental Epidemiology*, vol. 25, no. 1, pp. 37–44, 2013.

[GAN 82] GANDHI O.P., "Electromagnetic absorption in an inhomogeneous model of man for realistic exposure conditions", *Bioelectromagnetics*, vol. 3, no. 1, pp. 81–90, 1982.

[GAN 96] GANDHI O.P., LAZZI G., FURSE C.M., "Electromagnetic absorption in the human head and neck for mobile telephones at 835 and 1900 MHz", *IEEE Transactions on Microwave Theory and Techniques*, vol. 44, no. 10, pp. 1884–1897, 1996.

[GAT 09] GATI A., HADJEM A., WONG M.-F. *et al.*, "Exposure induced by WCDMA mobiles phones in operating networks", *IEEE Transactions on Wireless Communications*, vol. 8, no. 12, 2009.

[GHA 13] GHANMI A., Analyse de l'exposition aux ondes électromagnétiques des enfants dans le cadre des nouveaux usages et nouveaux réseaux, PhD Thesis, Université Marne La Vallée, 2013.

[GHA 14] GHANMI A., VARSIER N., HADJEM A. *et al.*, "Analysis of the influence of handset phone position on RF exposure of brain tissue", *Bioelectromagnetics*, vol. 35, no. 8, pp. 568–579, 2014.

[GHA 91] GHANEM R.G., SPANOS P., *Stochastic Finite Elements: A Spectral Approach*, Springer-Verlag, New York, 1991.

[GIL 00] GILLES L., HAGNESS S.C., VAZQUEZ L., "Comparison between staggered and unstaggered finite-difference time-domain grids for few-cycle temporal optical soliton propagation", *Journal of Computational Physics*, vol. 161, pp. 379–400, 2000.

[GOS 11a] GOSSELIN M.-C., KÜHN S., CRESPO-VALERO P. *et al.*, "Estimation of head-tissue specific exposure from mobile phones based on measurements in the homogeneous SAM head", *Bioelectromagnetics*, vol. 32, no. 6, pp. 493–505, 2011.

[GOS 11b] GOSSELIN M.-C., VERMEEREN G., KÜHN S. *et al.*, "Estimation formulas for the specific absorption rate in humans exposed to based stations antennas", *IEEE Transactions on Electromagnetic Compatibility*, vol. 53, no. 4, pp. 909–922, 2011.

[GOS 14] GOSSELIN M.-C., NEUFELD E., MOSER H. *et al.*, "Development of a new generation of high-resolution anatomical models for medical device evaluation: the Virtual Population 3.0", *Phys. Med. Biol.*, vol. 59, p. 5287, 2014.

[GRA 03] GRANGEA C., PERSON C., PICARD D. *et al.*, "Mesure du débit d'absorption spécifique (DAS) des téléphones mobiles", *Annales des Télécommunications*, vol. 58, no. 5/6, pp. 740–765, 2003.

[GUI 12] GUIFFAUT C., REINEIX A., PECQUEUX B., "New oblique thin wire formalism in the FDTD method with multiwire junctions", *IEEE Transactions on Antenna and Propagation*, vol. 60, no. 3, pp. 1458–1466, 2012.

[HAD 05] HADJEM A., LAUTRU D., DALE C. *et al.*, "Study of specific absorption rate (SAR) induced in the two child head models and adult heads using a mobile phones", *IEEE Transactions on Microwave Theory and Techniques*, vol. 53, pp. 4–11, 2005.

[HAN 88] HANSEN J., *Spherical Near-Field Antenna Measurements*, Peter Peregrinus Ltd., London, 1988.

[HAR 68] HARRINGTON R.F., *Field Computation by Moment Methods*, MacMillan, New York, 1968.

[HIR 08] HIRATA A., ITO N., FUJIWARA O. *et al.* "Conservative estimation of whole-body-averaged SARs in infants with a homogeneous and simple-shaped phantom in the GHz region", *Physics in Medicine and Biology,* vol. 53, no. 24, pp. 7215–7223, 2008.

[HOL 81] HOLLAND R., SIMPSON L., "Finite-difference analysis of EMP coupling to thin struts and wires", *IEEE Transactions on Electromagnetic Compatibility,* vol. 23, no. 2, pp. 88–97, 1981.

[HOL 83] HOLLAND R., WILLIAMS J.W., "Total field versus scattered field finite difference codes: a comparative assessment", *IEEE Transactions on Nuclear Science*, vol. 30, no. 6, pp. 4583, 1983.

[HUA 16] HUANG Y., NIKSIC S., KOCAN E. *et al.*, "Comparison of the average global exposure of the population induced by a macro 3G network in different geographical areas in France, Serbia and Montenegro", *Bioelectromagnetism*, 2016.

[HUT 79] HUTTENLOCHER P.R., "Synaptic density in human frontal cortex developmental changes and effects of aging", *Brain Research,* vol. 163, pp. 195–205, 1979.

[HWA 76] HWANG J.M.L., SHOUP R.L., POSTON J.W., "Mathematical description of a one- and five-year-old child for use in dosimetry calculations", Oak Ridge National Laboratory, Oak Ridge TN, 1976.

[ICN 98] ICNIRP, "Guidelines for limiting exposure to time-varying electric, magnetic and electromagnetic fields (up to 300 GHZ)", *Health Physics*, vol. 74, no. 4, pp. 494–522, 1998.

[ICT 14] ICT "Facts and figures", available at: https://www.itu.int/en/ITU-D/Statistics/Documents/facts/ICTFactsFigures2014-e.pdf, 2014.

[IEE 05] IEEE, Standard for safety levels with respect to human exposure to radio frequency electromagnetic fields, 3 kHz to 300 GHz, C95.1–2005, 2005.

[IEE 15a] IEEE, Determining the peak spatial-average specific absorption rate (SAR) in the human body from wireless communications devices: specific requirements for using the finite difference time domain (FDTD) method for SAR calculations of mobile phones, P 62704–3, 2015.

[IEE 15b] IEEE, Recommended practice for determining the peak spatial-average specific absorption rate (SAR) in the human body from wireless communications devices, 30 MHz – 6 GHz: specific requirements for finite difference time domain (FDTD), P 1528.3, 2015.

[JAL 14] JALA M., LÉVY-LEDUC C., MOULINES É. *et al.*, "Sequential design of computer experiments for the assessment of fetus exposure to electromagnetic fields", *Technometrics*, 2014.

[JAW 12] JAWAD O., LAUTRU D., BENLARBI-DELA A. *et al.*, "A human body model exposed to a cluster of waves: a statistical study of SAR", *Progress in Electromagnetics Research*, vol. 30, pp. 1–13, 2012.

[JAW 14] JAWAD O., LAUTRU D., BENLARBI-DELAI A. *et al.* "Study of human exposure using Kriging method", *Progress In Electromagnetics Research*, vol. 61, pp. 241–252, 2014.

[JEN 04] JENSEN F., AKSEL F., "On the number of modes in spherical wave expansions", *Proc. 26th AMTA*, Stone Mountain Park, GA, pp. 489–494, 2004.

[JOS 12] JOSEPH W. FREI P., RÖÖSLI M. *et al.*, "Between-country comparison of whole-body SAR from personal exposure data in urban areas", *Bioelectromagnetics*, vol. 33, no. 8, 2012.

[KAI 05] KAINZ W., CHRIST A., KELLOM T. *et al.*, "Dosimetric comparison of the specific anthropomorphic mannequin (SAM) to 14 anatomical head models using a novel definition for the mobile phone positioning", *Physics in Medicine and Biology*, vol. 50, no. 14, pp. 3423–3445, 2005.

[KEL 11] KELSH M.A., "Measured radiofrequency exposure during various mobile-phone use scenarios", *Journal of Exposure Science and Environmental Epidemiology*, vol. 21, pp. 343–354, 2011.

[KER 14] KERSAUDY P., MOSTARSHEDI S., SUDRET B. *et al.*, "Stochastic analysis of scattered field by building facades using polynomial chaos", *IEEE Transactions on Antenna & Propagation*, vol. 62, no. 12, pp. 6382–6393, 2014.

[KER 15] KERSAUDY P., SUDRET B., VARSIER N. *et al.*, "A new surrogate modeling technique combining Kriging and polynomial chaos expansions – application to uncertainty analysis in computational dosimetry", *Journal of Computational Physics*, vol. 286, pp. 103–117, 1 April 2015.

[KIE 11] KIENTEGA T., CONIL E., HADJEM A. *et al.*, "A surrogate model to assess the whole body SAR induced by multiple plane waves at 2.4 GHz", *Annals of Telecommunication*, vol. 66, pp. 419–428, 2011.

[KIM 08] KIM C.H., CHOI S.H., JEONG J.H. *et al.*, "HDRK-man: a whole body voxel model based on high resolution color slice images of a Korean adult male cadaver", *Physics in Medicine and Biology,* vol. 53, pp. 4093–4106, 2008.

[KRA 16] KRAYNI A., HADJEM A.H., SIBILLE A. *et al.*, "Analysis of the variability of the emitted power induced by personal device from numerical exposure simulations", *IEEE EMC*, 2016.

[KUC 12] KUCHERENKO S., TANRANTOLA S., ANNONI P., "Estimation of global sensitivity indices for models with dependent variables", *Computer Physics Communications*, vol. 183, pp. 937–946, 2012.

[KUN 93] KUNZ K., LUEBBER R., *The Finite Difference Time Domain Method for Electromagnetics*, CRC Press, New York, 1993.

[KUS 04] KUSTER N., SCHUDERER J., CHRIST A. *et al.*, "Guidance for exposure design of human studies addressing health risk evaluations of mobile phones", *Bioelectromagnetics*, vol. 25, no. 7, pp. 524–529, 2004.

[LAI 06] LAIHO J., WACKER A., NOVOSAD T., *Radio Network Planning and Optimisation for UMTS*, John Wiley and Sons Ltd, Chichester, 2006.

[LAR 05] LARCHEVÊQUE E., DALE C., WONG M.F. *et al.*, "Analysis of electric field averaging for in situ radiofrequency exposure assessment", *IEEE Transactions on Vehicular Technology*, vol. 52, no.4, pp. 1245–1250, 2005.

[LAU 00] LAUTRU D., Modélisation d'antennes filaires dans un maillage aux différences finies à l'aide d'une hybridation avec la méthode des moments dans le domaine temporel. Application à la dosimétrie des stations de base, PhD Thesis, University UMPC, Paris, 2000.

[LAU 01] LAUTRU D., WIART J., TABARRA W., "Analysis of thin wire antennas using a hybrid FDTD-MOMTD approach", *Annales des Télécommunications*, vol. 56, nos. 1–2, pp. 85–93, 2001.

[LEE 06] LEE A.K., CHOI W.Y., CHUNG M.S. *et al.* "Development of Korean male body model for computational dosimetry", *ETRI Journal,* vol. 28, pp. 107–110, 2006.

[LEE 07] LEE C., LODWICK D., HASENAUER D. *et al.* "Hybrid computational phantoms of the male and female newborn patient: NURBS-based whole-body models", *Physics in Medicine and Biology,* vol. 52, no. 12, pp. 3309–3333, 2007.

[LEE 09] LEE A.-K., BYUN J.-K., PARK J.S. *et al.*, "Development of 7-year-old Korean child model for computational dosimetry", *ETRI Journal*, vol. 31, no. 2, pp. 237–239, 2009.

[LEE 10] LEE C., LODWICK D., HURTADO J. *et al.*, "The UF family of reference hybrid phantoms for computational radiation dosimetry", *Physics in Medicine and Biology,* vol. 55, pp. 339–363, 2010.

[LEX 12] LEXNET, European Project, available at: www.lexnet-project.eu, 2012.

[LI 15] LI C., CHEN Z., YANG L. *et al.*, "Generation of infant anatomical models for evaluating the electromagnetic fields exposure", *Bioelectromagnetics*, vol. 36, no. 1, pp. 10–26, 2015.

[LON 05] LONN S., AHLBOM A., HALL P. *et al.*, "Long-term mobile phone use and brain tumor risk", *Am. J. Epidemiology*, vol. 161, no. 6, pp. 526–535, 2005.

[MAH 11] MAHFOUZ Z., GATI A., LAUTRU D. *et al.*, "Influence of traffic variations on exposure to wireless signals in realistic environements", *Bioelectromagnetics*, vol. 33, pp. 288–297, 2011.

[MAH 12] MAHFOUZ Z., Analyse de l'exposition aux ondes électromagnétiques en Indoor, PhD Thesis, University UPMC Paris VI, 2012.

[MAX 04] MAXWELL J.C., *A Treatise on Electricity and Magnetism*, 3rd ed., vol 1, Clarendon Press, Oxford, 1904.

[MAX 65] MAXWELL J.C., "A dynamical theory of the electromagnetic field", *Royal Society Transactions*, vol. 155, pp. 459–512, 1865.

[MC 79] MCKAY M.D., CONOVER W.J., BECKMAN R.J., "A comparison of three methods for selecting values of input variables in the analysis of output from a computer code", *Technometrics*, vol. 21, pp. 239–245, 1979.

[MER 80] MEREWETHER D.E., FISHER R., SMITH F.W., "On implementing a numeric Huygen's source in a finite difference program to illuminate scattering bodies", *IEEE Transactions on Nuclear Science*, vol. 27, no. 6, pp. 1829–1833, 1980.

[MIL 73] MILLER E.K., POGGIO A.J., BURKE G.J., "An integro-differential equation technique for the time-domain analysis of thin wire structures", *Journal of Computational Physics*, vol. 12, no.1, pp. 24–48, 1973.

[MON 03] MONEBHURRUN V., DALE C., BOLOMEY J.C. *et al.*, "A numerical approach for the determination of the tissue equivalent liquid used during SAR assessment", *IEEE Transactions on Magnetics*, vol. 38, no. 2, pp. 745–748, 2003.

[MOS 10] MOSTARSHEDI S., RICHALOT E., LAHEURTE J.-M. *et al.*, "Fast and accurate calculation of scattered EM fields from building faces using Green's functions of semi-infinite medium", *IET Microwaves, Antennas & Propagation*, vol. 4, no. 1, pp.72–82, 2010.

[MOS 84] MOSIG J.R., Les structures microruban: analyse au moyen des équations intégrales, PhD Thesis, Ecole Polytechnique Fédérale de Lausanne, 1984.

[MUR 81] MUR G., "Absorbing boundary conditions for the finite difference approximation of the time-domain electromagnetic-field equations", *IEEE Transactions on Electromagnetic Compatibility*, vol. 23, no. 4, pp. 377–382, 1981.

[NAG 04] NAGAOKA T., WATANABE S., SAKURAI K. *et al.*, "Development of realistic high resolution whole-body voxel models of Japanese adult male and female of average height and weight, and application of models to radio-frequency electromagnetic-field dosimetry", *Physics in Medicine and Biology*, vol. 49, pp. 1–15, 2004.

[NAG 07] NAGAOKA T., TOGASHI T., SAITO K. *et al.*, "Anatomically realistic whole-body pregnant-woman model and specific absorption rates for pregnant-woman exposure to electromagnetic plane waves from 10 MHz to 2 GHz", *Physics in Medicine and Biology*, vol. 52, no. 22, pp. 6731–6743, 2007.

[NAG 08] NAGAOKA T., KUNIEDA E., WATANABE S., "Proportion-corrected scaled voxel models for Japanese children and their application to the numerical dosimetry of specific absorption rate for frequencies from 30 MHz to 3 GHz", *Physics in Medicine and Biology*, vol. 53, pp. 6695–6711, 2008.

[NAT 62] NATAF A., "Détermination des distributions dont les marges sont données", *C.R. de l'Académie des Sciences*, vol. 225, pp. 42–43, 1962.

[NIC 01] NICOLAS E., LAUTRU D., JACQUIN F. *et al.*, "Specific absorption rate assessment based on a selective isotropic measuring system for electromagnetic field", *IEEE Transactions on Instrumentation and Measurements*, vol. 50, no. 2, pp. 397–401, 2001.

[OKO 97] OKONIEWSKI M., OKONIEWSKA E., STUCHLY M., "Three-dimensional sub gridding algorihtm for FDTD", *IEEE Transactionson Antennas and Propagation*, vol. 45, pp. 422–429, 1997.

[OUL 07] OULD ISSELMOU Y., Interpolation spatiale de niveaux d'exposition aux émissions radioélectriques in situ à l'aide de méthodes géostatistiques, PhD Thesis, Ecoles des Mines de Paris, 2007.

[OUL 08] OULD ISSELMOU Y., WACKERNAGEL H., TABBARA W. *et al.* "Geostatistical estimation of electromagnetic exposure", in SOARES A., PEREIRA M., DIMITRAKOPOULOS R. (eds), *Geostatistics for Environmental Applications*, Springer, 2008.

[PAR 05] PARK, J.S., CHUNG, M.S., HWANG, S.B. *et al.*, "Visible Korean human: improved serially sectioned images of the entire body", *IEEE Transaction on Medical Imaging*, vol. 24, no. 3, pp. 352–360, 2005.

[PAS 07] PASCAUD R., GILLARD R., LIOSON R., "A dual-grid FDTD scheme for the fast simulation of surrounded antennas", *IET Microwaves, Antennas & Propagation*, vol. 1, no. 3, pp. 700–706, 2007.

[PET 02] PETOUSSI-HENSS N., ZANKI M., FILL U. *et al.* "The GSF family of voxel phantoms", *Physics in Medicine and Biology,* vol. 47, no. 1, pp. 89–106, 2002.

[PET 98] PETOUSSI-HENSS N., ZANKL M., "Voxel anthropomorphic models as a tool for internal dosimetry", *Radiation Protection Dosimetry*, vol. 79, pp. 415–418, 1998.

[PIN 11] PINTO Y., GHANMI A., HADJEM A. e*t al.*, "Numerical mobile phone models validated by SAR measurements", *5th European Conference on Antennas and Propagation*, pp. 2585–2588, Rome, Italy, April 2011.

[POK 00] POKOVIC K., SCHMID T., FRÖHLICH J. *et al.* "Novel probes and evaluation procedures to assess field magnitude and polarization", *IEEE Transactions on Electromagnetic Compatibility*, vol. 42, no. 2, pp. 240–244, 2000.

[PRA 06] PRADIER A., LACROUX F., LAUTRU D. e*t al.* "SAR assessment using tissues homogenization technique", *Proceedings EuCAP*, Nice, France. pp 1–4, November 2006.

[PRA 08a] PRADIER A., HADJEM A., LAUTRU D. *et al.* "Evaluation of the SAR induced in a multilayer biological structure and comparison with SAR in homogeneous tissues", *Annals of Telecommunications*, vol. 63, pp. 79–86, 2008.

[PRA 08b] PRADIER T., Evaluation des champs électromagnétiques induits dans les tissus biologiques pour les nouveaux usages et les nouvelles technologies sans fil, PhD Thesis, University UPMC Paris VI, 2008.

[QIA 09] QIAN P.Z.G., "Nested Latin hypercube designs", *Biometrika*, vol. 96, no. 4, pp. 957–970, 2009.

[RAM 97] RAMAHI O.M., "Near- and far-field calculations in FDTD simulations using Kirchhoff surface integral representation", *IEEE Transactions on Antennas Propagation*, vol. 45, no. 5, 1997.

[REN 00] RENGARAJAN S.R., RAHMAT-SAMII, Y., "The field equivalence principle: illustration of the establishment of the non-intuitive null fields", *IEEE Transactions on Antenna and Propagation,* vol. 42, no. 4, pp. 122–128, 2000.

[ROS 00] ROSSI J.-P., WIART J., EYNARD F., "In situ measurement of building reflection and diffraction coefficients of UHF radio-waves using a ring array", *Radiosciences*, vol. 35, no. 2, pp. 361–369, 2000.

[ROS 52] ROSENBLATT M., "Remarks on a multivariate transformation", *Annals of Mathematical Statistics*, vol. 23, pp. 470–472, 1952.

[SAC 95] SACKS Z.S., KINGSLAND D.M., LEE R. *et al.*, "A perfectly matched anisotropic absorber for use as an absorbing boundary condition", *IEEE Transactions on Antennas and Propagation*, vol. 43, no. 12, pp. 1460–1463, 1995.

[SAI 08] SAIDI F., LAUTRU D., GATI A. *et al.*, "An on-site SAR evaluation using interpolation and plane-wave decomposition", *IEEE Microwave and Optical Technology Letters*, vol. 50, no. 6, pp. 1501–1505, 2008.

[SAL 00] SALTELLI A., CHAN K., SCOTT E. (eds), *Sensitivity Analysis*, John Wiley & Sons, Oxford, 2000.

[SCH 11] SCHÜZ J., ELLIOTT P., AUVINENC A. *et al.*, "An international prospective cohortstudy of mobile phone users and health (Cosmos): Design considerations and enrolment", *Cancer Epidemiology*, vol. 35, no. 1, pp. 37–43, February 2011.

[SCH 96] SCHMID T., EGGER O., KUSTER N., "Automated E-field scanning system for dosimetric assessments", *IEEE Transactions on Microwave Theory and Techniques*, vol. 44, no. 1, pp. 105–113, 1996.

[SCH 98] SCHOENBORN F., BURHARDT V., KUSTER N., "Difference in energy absorption between heads of adults and children in the near field of sources". *Health Physics*, vol. 74, pp. 160–168, 1998.

[SHA 49] SHANNON C., "Communication theory of secrecy systems", *Bell System Technical Journal*, vol. 28, no. 4, pp. 656–715, 1949.

[SHL 95] SHLAGER K.L., SMITH S., "Comparison of two FDTD near-field to near-field transformations applied to pulsed antenna problems", *Electronic Letters*, vol. 31, no. 12, pp. 936–938, 1995.

[SHO 00] SHOUTENS W., *Stochastic Processes and Orthogonal Polynomials*, Springer-Verlag, New York, 2000.

[SIL 08] SILLY-CARETTE J., LAUTRU D., GATI A. *et al.*, "Optimisation of the homogenization of tissues using the adjoint method and the FDTD", *IEEE MTT-S International*, Atlanta, GA, pp. 1361–1364 June 2008

[SIL 09] SILLY-CARETTE J., LAUTRU D., WONG M.F. *et al.*, "Variability on the propagation of a plane wave using stochastic collocation methods in a bio electromagnetic application", *IEEE Microwave and Wireless Components Letters*, vol. 19, no. 4, 185–187, 2009.

[SMO 63] SMOLYAK S., "Quadrature and interpolation formulas for tensor products of certain classes of functions", *Soviet Mathematics Doklady*, vol. 4, pp. 240–243, 1963.

[SOB 93] SOBOL I.M., "Sensitivity estimates for nonlinear mathematical models", *Math. Model & Comput. Exp.*, vol. 1, no. 4, pp. 407–414, 1993.

[SOI 04] SOIZE C., GHANEM R., "Physical systems with random uncertainties: chaos representations with arbitrary probability measure", *SIAM Journal on Scientific Computing*, vol. 26, no. 2, pp. 395–410, 2004.

[STR 41] STRATTON J.A., *Electromagnetic Theory*, Mc Graw-Hill, New York,1941.

[SUD 07] SUDRET B., Uncertainty propagation and sensitivity analysis in mechanical models. Contribution to structural reliability and stochastic spectral method, Thesis, available at http://www.ibk.ethz.ch/ su/publications/Reports/ HDRSudret.pdf, University Blaise Pascal, Clermont-Ferrand, France, 2007.

[TAV 95] TAFLOVE A., *Computational Electrodynamics, The Finite Difference Time Domain Metho*, Artech House, Boston, 1995.

[TES 14] TESANOVIC M., CONIL E., DE DOMENICO A. *et al.*, "The LEXNET project: wireless networks and emf: paving the way for low-emf networks of the future", *Vehicular Technology Magazine IEEE*, vol. 9, no. 2, pp. 20–28 May 2014.

[TIB 96] TIBSHIRANI R., "Regression shrinkage and selection via the Lasso", *Journal of Royal Statistical Society, Series B*, vol. 58, pp. 267–288, 1996.

[TRO 08] TROISI F. *et al.*, "The Italian national electromagnetic field monitoring network", *Annals Telecommunication*, vol. 63, pp. 97–108, 2008.

[VAL 02] VALENTIN J., "Basic anatomical and physiological data for use in radiological protection: reference values", *Annals of the ICRP*, vol. 32, pp. 1–277, September 2002.

[VAR 14] VARSIER N., DAHDOUH S., SERRURIER A. *et al.*, "Influence of pregnancy stage and fetus position on the whole-body and local exposure of the fetus to RF-EMF", *Physics in Medicine and Biology*, vol. 59, no. 17, p. 4913, 2014.

[VAR 15] VARSIER E.I., "A novel method to assess the human population exposure induced by a wireless telecommunication network", *Bioelectromagnetics*, vol. 36, no. 6, pp. 451–463, September 2015.

[VER 10] VERMEEREN G., GOSSELIN M.C., KUHN S. *et al.*, "The influence of the reflective environment on the absorption of a human male exposed to representative base station antennas from 300 MHz to 5 GHz", *Physics in Medicine and Biology*, vol. 55, pp. 5541–5555, 2010.

[VIE 09] VIEL J.F. *et al.*, "Residential exposure to radiofrequency fields from mobile phone base stations, and broadcast transmitters: a population-based survey with personal meter", *Occupational and Environmental Medicine*, vol. 66, no. 8, pp. 550–556, 2009.

[VRI 09] VRIJHEID M., MANN S., VECCHAI P. *et al.*, "Determinants of mobile phone output power in a multinational study: implications for exposure assessment", *Occupational and Environmental Medicine*, vol. 66, no. 10, pp. 664–671, 2009.

[WAI 96] WAIT J.R. *et al.*, *Electromagnetic Waves in Stratified Media*, IEEE, 1996.

[WAN 03a] WANG G.G., "Adaptive response surface method using inherited latin hypercube design points", *Journal of Mechanical Design*, vol. 125, pp. 210–220, 2003.

[WAN 03b] WANG J., FUJIWARA O., "Comparison and evaluation of electromagnetic absorption characteristics in realistic children for 900-MHz mobile telephones", *IEEE Transactions on Microwave Theory and Techniques*, vol. 51 pp. 966–71, 2003.

[WIA 95] WIART J., Propagation des ondes radioélectriques en milieu urbain dans un contexte microcellulaire. analyse par la gtd et validation expérimentale, Thesis, Univeristy Paris VI, 1995.

[WIA 98] WIART J, MITTRA R, CHAILLOU S. *et al.*, "The analysis of human head interaction with a hand-held mobile using the non-uniform FDTD", *IEEE APS Conference on Antennas and Propagation for Wireless Communications*, Waltham, MA, 1998.

[WIA 00] WIART J. DALE C., BOSISIO A.V. *et* al., "Analysis of the influence of the power control and discontinuous transmission on RF exposure with GSM mobile phones", *IEEE Transactions on Electromagnetic Compatibility*, vol. 42, no. 2, pp. 376–384, 2000.

[WIA 01] WIART J., "Electromagnétisme appliqué à la dosimétrie des interactions des ondes radioélectrique avec les personnes", *Communication Mobile. Effets Biologiques*, Editions Tec&Doc, pp. 5–28, 2001.

[WIA 05] WIART J., HADJEM A., GADI N. *et al.* "Modeling of RF exposure in children", *Bioelectromagnetics*, vol. 26, no. S7, pp. 45–50, 2005.

[WIA 08] WIART J. *et al.*, "Analysis of RF exposure in the head tissues of children and adults", *Physics in Medicine and Biology,* vol. 53, pp. 3681–3695, 2008.

[WIA 11] WIART J. *et al.*, "Numerical dosimetry dedicated to children RF exposure", *Progress in Biophysics and Molecular Biology*, vol. 107, no. 3, pp. 421–427, 2011.

[WIA 15] WIART J., KERSAUDY P., GHANMI A. *et al.* "Stochastic dosimetry to manage uncertainty in numerical EMF exposure assessment", *Forum for Electromagnetic Research Methods and Application Technologies*, vol. 12, 2015.

[WIE 38] WIENER N., "The homogeneous chaos", *American Journal of Mathematics*, vol. 60, pp. 897–936, 1938.

[WON 00] WONG M.F., FOUAD HANNA V., WIART J. *et al.*, "Finite element formulation of space-time subgridding scheme in the FDTD method", *International Journal of Numerical Modeling*, vol. 13, nos. 2–3, pp.127–137, 2000.

[WON 95] WONG M.F., PICON O., FOUAD HANNA V., "A finite element method based on Whitney forms to solve Maxwell equations in the time domain", *IEEE Transition on Magnetics*, vol. 31, pp. 1618–1621, 1995.

[WU 11] WU T., TAN L., SHAO Q. *et al.*, "Chinese adult anatomical models and the application in evaluation of RF exposures", *Physics in Medicine and Biology*, vol. 56, pp. 2075–2089, 2011.

[XIU 05] XIU D., HESTHAVEN J., "High-order collocation methods for differential equations with random input", *SIAM Journal of Scientific Computing*, vol. 27, no. 3, pp. 1118–1139, 2005.

[XU 00] XU X.G., CHAO T.C., BOZKURT A., "VIP-MAN: an image based whole-body adult male model constructed from color photographs of the Visible Human Project for multi-particle Monte Carlo calculations", *Health Physics*, vol. 78, pp. 476–485, 2000.

[XU 10] XU X.G., ECKERMAN, K.F., *Handbook of Anatomical Models for Radiation Dosimetry Series in Medical Physics and Biomedical Engineering*, CRC Press, 2010.

[YEE 66] YEE K., "Numerical solution of initial boundary value problems involving Maxwell's equations in isotropic media", *IEEE Transactions on Antennas and Propagation*, vol. 16, pp. 302–307, 1966.

[ZAN 88] ZANKL M., VEIT R., WILLIAMS G. *et al.*, "The construction of computer tomographic phantoms and their application in radiology and radiation protection", *Radiation and Environmental Biophysics*, vol. 27, pp. 153–164, 1988.

[ZHA 05] ZHANG S.-X., HENG P.-A., LIU Z.-J., "Chinese visible human project: dataset acquisition and its primary applications", *Proceedings of the IEEE Engineering in Medicine and Biology 27th Annual Conference*, Shanghai, China, September 1–4 2005.

[ZUB 94] ZUBAL I.G. *et al.*, "Computerized 3D segmented human anatomy", *Med. Phy.*, vol. 21, pp. 299–302, 1994.

Index

Other titles from

iSTE

in

Waves

2016

ANSELMET Fabien, MATTEI Pierre-Olivier
Acoustics, Aeroacoustics and Vibrations

PARET Dominique
Antennas Designs for NFC Devices

2015

PICART Pascal
New Techniques in Digital Holography

2014

APPRIOU Alain
Uncertainty Theories and Multisensor Data Fusion

JARRY Pierre, BENEAT Jacques N.
RF and Microwave Electromagnetism

LAHEURTE Jean-Marc
UHF RFID Technologies for Identification and Traceability

SAVAUX Vincent, LOUËT Yves
MMSE-based Algorithm for Joint Signal Detection, Channel and Noise Variance Estimation for OFDM Systems

THOMAS Jean-Hugh, YAAKOUBI Nourdin
New Sensors and Processing Chain

TING Michael
Molecular Imaging in Nano MRI

VALIÈRE Jean-Christophe
Acoustic Particle Velocity Measurements using Laser: Principles, Signal Processing and Applications

VANBÉSIEN Olivier, CENTENO Emmanuel
Dispersion Engineering for Integrated Nanophotonics

2013

BENMAMMAR Badr, AMRAOUI Asma
Radio Resource Allocation and Dynamic Spectrum Access

BOURLIER Christophe, PINEL Nicolas, KUBICKÉ Gildas
Method of Moments for 2D Scattering Problems: Basic Concepts and Applications

GOURE Jean-Pierre
Optics in Instruments: Applications in Biology and Medicine

LAZAROV Andon, KOSTADINOV Todor Pavlov
Bistatic SAR/GISAR/FISAR Theory Algorithms and Program Implementation

LHEURETTE Eric
Metamaterials and Wave Control

PINEL Nicolas, BOURLIER Christophe
Electromagnetic Wave Scattering from Random Rough Surfaces: Asymptotic models

SHINOHARA Naoki
Wireless Power Transfer via Radiowaves

TERRE Michel, PISCHELLA Mylène, VIVIER Emmanuelle
Wireless Telecommunication Systems

2012

LALAUZE René
Chemical Sensors and Biosensors

LE MENN Marc
Instrumentation and Metrology in Oceanography

LI Jun-chang, PICART Pascal
Digital Holography

2011

BECHERRAWY Tamer
Mechanical and Electromagnetic Vibrations and Waves

GROUS Ammar
Applied Metrology for Manufacturing Engineering

GOURE Jean-Pierre
Optics in Instruments

LE CHEVALIER François, LESSELIER Dominique, STARAJ Robert
Non-standard Antennas

2010

BEGAUD Xavier
Ultra Wide Band Antennas

MARAGE Jean-Paul, MORI Yvon
Sonar and Underwater Acoustics

2009

BOUDRIOUA Azzedine
Photonic Waveguides

BRUNEAU Michel, POTEL Catherine
Materials and Acoustics Handbook

DE FORNEL Frederique, FAVENNEC Pierre-Noël
Measurements using Optic and RF Waves

FRENCH COLLEGE OF METROLOGY
Transverse Disciplines in Metrology

2008

FILIPPI Paul J.T.
Vibrations and Acoustic Radiation of Thin Structures

LALAUZE René
Physical Chemistry of Solid-Gas Interfaces

2007

KUNDU Tribikram
Advanced Ultrasonic Methods for Material and Structure Inspection

PLACKO Dominique
Fundamentals of Instrumentation and Measurement

RIPKA Pavel, TIPEK Alois
Modern Sensors Handbook

2006

BALAGEAS Daniel *et al.*
Structural Health Monitoring

BOUCHET Olivier *et al.*
Free-Space Optics

BRUNEAU Michel, SCELO Thomas
Fundamentals of Acoustics

FRENCH COLLEGE OF METROLOGY
Metrology in Industry

GUILLAUME Philippe
Music and Acoustics

GUYADER Jean-Louis
Vibration in Continuous Media

Lightning Source UK Ltd.
Milton Keynes UK
UKOW06n1419190416

272550UK00001B/4/P

9 781848 218567

Pn